OXFORD MED

Surgery for (

Surgery for General Practitioners

Brian A. Maurice MA, MCHir, FRCS

Formerly Consultant Surgeon
Kent and Sussex Hospital
Tunbridge Wells, UK and
Surgical Tutor to the
Royal College of Surgeons

Oxford New York Tokyo
OXFORD UNIVERSITY PRESS

Oxford University Press, Walton Street, Oxford OX2 6DP
Oxford New York Toronto
Delhi Bombay Calcutta Madras Karachi
Kuala Lumpur Singapore Hong Kong Tokyo
Nairobi Dar es Salaam Cape Town
Melbourne Auckland Madrid
and associated companies in
Berlin Ibadan

Oxford is a trade mark of Oxford University Press

Published in the United States by
Oxford University Press Inc., New York

First published in 1989 by
Castle House Publications Ltd
Tunbridge Wells, Kent

Reprinted 1992 (with corrections), 1993

British Library Cataloguing in Publication Data
Maurice, Brian A.
Surgery for General Practitioners
1. Medicine. Surgery. Operations. Manuals
I. Title
617.'91

ISBN 0–7194–0136–4

Library of Congress Cataloging in Publication Data
(Data available on request)

ISBN 0–7194–0136–4

Illustrations by Shona Grant, Reigate, Surrey
Printed in Great Britain by
The Ipswich Book Company, Ipswich, Suffolk

Dosages and other such information have been included in this publication. Despite careful checking, mistakes may have occurred and any such information should be checked with the package insert, British National Formulary, or other suitable reference source.

Contents

Preface

Having been present at the conception of the ideas for this book when Brian Maurice started his talks on Surgery in General Practice for our Tunbridge Wells trainees, it is a pleasure to recommend it now.

Honed and clarified by his experience of the trainees' needs and the ideas of his many General Practice friends, this is essentially a practical book for the General Practitioner who is thinking of starting surgery after years of allowing his surgical skills to lie fallow. It is also for the General Practitioner who is keen to improve his technique.

There are sensible, economic suggestions for setting up a theatre and putting together equipment, as well as chapters on documentation, sterilisation, cutting style, good stitchcraft, and wise recommendations for consent forms. The chapter on local anaesthesia by Berwyn Thomas will help us all towards better pain-free work. Additionally, there are excellent chapters on more specific procedures which are simply and vividly presented. This will give the average and not-too-adventurous General Practitioner the necessary preparation to embark on a very satisfying surgical voyage.

With the impending Government review of the National Health Service funding and expected implementation of the White Paper on Primary Care, I might say that the financial rewards will give greater opportunity for General Practitioners to take up the ideas in this book. Health Authority managers, put into an internal market and under pressure to find money-saving outlets, will look to General Practice to offer an economic alternative for some surgery in their Districts.

So, it is with pleasure that I commend this book to all my General Practice friends and colleagues, both trainees and trainers, and both young and old.

A. J. Membrey MB, FRCGP
General Practitioner, Tunbridge Wells
Examiner for the Membership of the Royal College of General Practioners
Member of the Council of the Royal College of General Practitioners 1984 to 1987

1989

To my wife Sammy and our children Adrian, Laura and Christopher. For all their love and understanding, ever hoping,

MOLIRI EST VINCERE

CHAPTER 1

Introduction

This book is based on some occasional postgraduate lectures with the theme 'Surgery in your Surgeries' given to general practitioners and postgraduate vocational training courses. Following the ensuing discussions and due to their encouragement and enthusiasm this book is now produced.

The general practitioner or family doctor in the U.K. at the present time is gradually altering from one who is in practice by himself to the development of the group practice and multiple partnership usually operating from one large surgery or, in some cases, from a medical centre specifically designed for the purpose.

These partnerships have secretarial and lay staff to provide the back-up administrative support for the doctors to enable the practice to run smoothly. Nursing personnel are available either full or part time, working both in the medical centre or visiting patients in their homes.

A partnership with the practice being shared means that there is an opportunity for each of the individuals in the group to develop their own skills and particular interests. Amongst them are some who, after qualification, perhaps initially considered attempting to specialise in one of the surgical disciplines in hospital practice but who subsequently decided that the future vehicle for their own talents and skill lay in general practice.

Surgery gives its satisfaction in two ways to those who practise it. Firstly, the stimulus from the challenge of the difficult diagnostic problem presented and overcome, and secondly, the aesthetic pleasure of performing a technical operation well — to the ultimate satisfaction of the patient and the surgeon alike.

In a sophisticated society there is no place for a general practitioner to do the occasional minor operation in his surgery with conditions which are unsuitable; with a technique that is untried; and support facilities which leave much to be desired.

Equally, there is a very real place for one partner of a group practice, who is interested in the technical side of surgery, to perform minor operations in a well organised set-up at regular intervals, doing a list of all his own minor surgery and, one assumes, those of his colleagues in the partnership that have been referred to him.

The diagnostic challenge in this kind of surgical practice may be small, but the challenge to perform a beautiful, technical procedure is a very real one and the satisfaction derived from it is commensurate with the quality of its execution.

This is not only stimulating for the general practitioner who is interested in the technical side of surgery, it is also very rewarding and provides a very much appreciated service for the patient. It saves the patient visits to local hospital out-patient clinics, saves them waiting for out-patient theatre time and usually, in the final analysis, it saves the operation being carried out by a junior doctor in the hospital on a patient he has never seen before.

Although in such a group practice there may be one member interested in doing the minor surgery, there may also be another partner who has an interest in anaesthesia and, indeed, might have had experience of this speciality before going into general practice.

Superficially it would seem to be a very good idea to be combining the talents of a doctor giving the general anaesthetic with the one performing the surgery. However, if this is to be done properly, without risk, the whole surgical and anaesthetic set-up would need enlarging. While this would widen the scope of the operations that could be undertaken, it would not increase the surgical repertoire sufficiently to justify the additional equipment, space and back-up personnel needed to make it safe and effective. The scope of this book, therefore, is limited to surgery which can be carried out under local anaesthetic.

Fortunately, some general practitioners with an interest in surgery can still do some minor surgery in local cottage hospitals which have not yet been closed down, and to which they have access.

This, however, is a relatively routine procedure as in cottage hospitals there are the nursing staff, the fabric of the theatre and sterilising areas, the instruments and organisation, all available and provided on the spot. Usually there is a fully trained theatre nurse to prepare, set up and assist at any of these procedures. To be able to undertake minor operations in the general practice surgery or medical centre, all the facilities available in cottage hospital theatres have to be planned and organised first.

Also, as the doctor may perhaps have the help of only an unqualified lay person, the organisation has to be arranged so that no detailed medical knowledge is needed for the initial preparation for any operation.

The first part of this book is devoted to planning the surgical area and suggestions for its organisation and running in a general practice situation.

The theatre preparation has been made as simple as possible so that if there is any doubt about what is needed, reference can be made to the appropriate chapter by the assistant. By using the system of 'unit packs' and standard instruments and drugs, it is hoped that confusion will be avoided and that the variation of set-up for differing procedures will be minimal and not too complicated.

Instruments and their varying designs and usage are discussed. Set out are the general principles of surgery and surgical management of tissue, followed by chapters on anaesthetic techniques and administration.

Trauma and infective conditions are discussed in the final chapters on the detailed description of the elective surgical procedures; these are described under their own particular headings.

Many patients who know their general practitioner personally and with confidence built up over the years, greatly prefer this type of minor surgery to be carried out by him.

If this confidence is not going to be misfounded everything must be done correctly and run smoothly from the moment the patient presents with the original problem until the final stitches are removed. This means detailed organisation and forethought so that at the end of the day there is not only a patient pleased with the result of the procedure, but also a surgeon with the satisfaction of a technical operation having been performed in a first-class manner.

CHAPTER 2

Operating Theatre, Set-up and Organisation

Surgery

In a general practice building, whether custom-built or not, it is unrealistic to suggest that a separate room should be put aside for sole use as a minor operating theatre. However, for the minor operating session to be carried out properly there are many principles that should be observed when arranging the actual hardwear of the theatre area.

The room

This should be of adequate size to allow free movement of two people, having made allowances for couches, store areas, prep areas, etc.

It should not be used as a through-way to get elsewhere when no surgery is taking place.

The floor

Preferably of a continuous washable surface.

The walls

Decorated, if possible, in a monochrome — either white for lightness or green for restfulness for the eyes.

The surface should be washable and all extraneous dust-collecting excrescences should be removed, i.e. curtain rails, old fireplaces and mantlepieces if still present in an old building.

Windows

As much natural light as possible should be allowed in.

When the window, of whatever make or design, is opened, the gap created should have insect-free net across it to keep out flies and wasps, etc.

The windows, which may need opaque glass for social reasons, should be able to be opened with the minimal amount of effort and without having to stretch across any vital clean area to reach them.

The door

Ideally it is a great help if the door has a glass window in its top half to enable anyone outside, in the rest of the surgery, to see what is happening inside without having to enter and disrupt an operation.

The door must be fitted with a self-closing spring.

Warning bells and lights

1. There must be a light on the outside of the door with its controlling switch inside which, when switched on, indicates that an operation is in progress.
2. There must be a bell in the main reception area of the office or in the secretary's office of the main building so that aid can be summoned in an emergency without the surgeon having to shout the full length of the building. This bell should be controlled by a foot switch on a block on the end of a cable which can be sited underneath the operating table and can always be within reach of the surgeon or assistant.
3. It is a great help sometimes to have an intercom if the medical centre is already fitted and wired for it.

Heating

Adequate heating is essential for both the patient and surgeon.

The type of heating will depend on that already installed, but a blower heater is not advised as it creates excessive turbulence and air currents which stir up dust and increase the risk of contamination.

Operating couch

Although an operating table with all its sophistication is ideal, it is probably impractical from the financial point of view and, therefore, an ordinary examination couch with plastic cover, over which there is a clean white sheet, should be adequate.

The difficulty with this is that the height is not variable, so it is important that the correct height is fixed at the outset when designing the surgery.

This height should be such that the patient's abdominal wall, when lying flat on his back on the couch, should be at the level of the surgeon's hands when his elbow is flexed at 90° and the upper arm vertical, i.e. the arms in the 'playing the piano' position.

The couch or table should also have a padded side limb arrangement on which to place the patient's arm when he is lying flat on his back, and the surgery is, for example, being carried out on his hand.

This, on a couch or table, will have to be added by means of a hinged flap which, when not in use, hangs down or can be detached. Alternatively, a mobile trolley of the correct height can be used alongside the couch. The disadvantage of this is that if the surgeon wishes to sit whilst operating on a hand, he is unable to put his legs under the trolley — this is not only uncomfortable but it is also bad technique to operate at a distance.

The best arrangement is a 20 cm to 23 cm broad flap, hinged on the side of the couch which, when lifted out, is supported by a leg which swings down from the hinge at its outer end.

Whichever method is used it must be:

1. Safe and firm, not only for the patient but also when any pressure is put on it by the surgeon.
2. Movable, so that it does not intrude when not needed.
3. Fully padded so that the patient's arm is comfortable when resting on it.

It is important to establish a proper facility for surgery on the arm and hand, if at all possible.

The practice of having the patient sitting on a chair with the hand on the couch seems, superficially, to be the answer, but if at any time during the procedure the patient feels faint then the whole performance becomes chaotic in a few seconds. The principle of having the patient flat and relaxed is an important one.

Position of operating table

Ideally, the table should be in the centre of the room with full access on all sides. If this is not possible, it could project from a wall from its head end, leaving access along both long sides and the foot.

On no account should access be less than that whilst surgery is taking place even if the table is pushed aside when not in use.

Lighting

1. *Natural light* as previously described.
2. *Everyday light* for the room, when surgery is not taking place, can be the normal free-hanging light from the ceiling, or wall lights as convenient.
3. *Operating light* The principle of a shadowless light is that the light source is, in fact, not one but multiple beams focusing from all around on to the area or field of operation thus getting under an intruding hand, leaving the underlying field well illuminated. (See Figure 2.1.)

   As a full purpose-built operating light is not envisaged there should be:

(a) At least two Anglepoise-type lamps with powerful bulbs which can shine in from different angles.
(b) Photoflood light in its own holders. These lamps are very powerful and have their own built-in reflectors and, for this reason, should be considered. However, as they are virtually unprotected they are at risk of being damaged.
(c) Mobile stand spotlights — these are manufactured as a specific entity of theatre equipment, are very efficient and one is a very helpful adjunct.

It is always to be remembered that if a surgery has too much light it can always be reduced by switching something off. If it has too little, increasing it at a moment's notice, becomes a major performance.

Siting of Anglepoise lamps

It is important, if possible, to have the lamps as a fixture rather than on various mobile stands. This makes for stability in positioning the light and for less clutter around the patient and table, making access easier. It also means that fewer things have to be moved from the floor for its cleaning.

It is difficult to be dogmatic about the siting of the lamps, but it should be remembered that they must be able to illuminate both the hand on an outstretched arm-board, and also the abdomen, scrotum or feet areas on the couch, for their respective surgery. Therefore, it is probably best to have a combination of two fixed Anglepoise-type lamps, one over the hand area and one over the central part of the couch, and combine these with one mobile spot lamp which can be moved to augment either of the previous two.

Figure 2.1 Siting of lamps

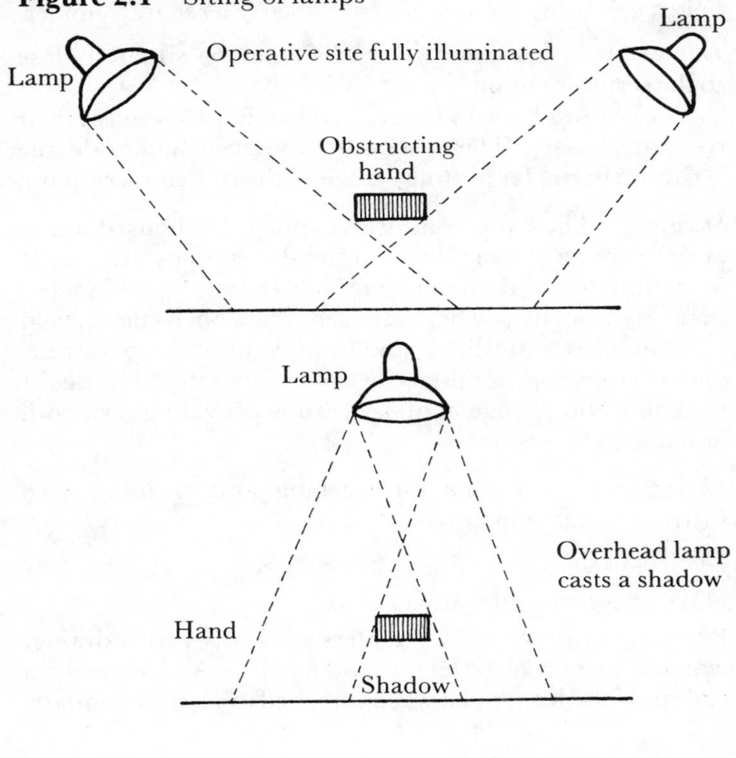

Wash-up arrangements

1. *Basin* The sink for the surgeon's wash and scrub-up, should be arranged so that there is a mixer tap installed with plenty of room beneath the tap and above the sink to make washing of hands and arms easy.

   The mixer should be a long-handled tap variety which enables the relative flow from hot and cold pipes to be adjusted and the taps switched on and off with the handles being manipulated by the surgeon's elbows, which are not clean.

2. *Soaps, etc.* If Hibiscrub or other such scrub-up antiseptic detergent is being used, the dispenser controlled by an elbow lever should be above the taps and basin.

   Soap trays should always be self-draining so as not to accumulate soapy water with its potential infection in the bottom of the receptacle. It should also be large enough to hold a nail brush if one is not contained in a separate holder.

3. *Hats and masks containers* These should be situated close to the scrub-up basin.

   The hats and masks mentioned in Chapter 4, have their own dispensers. These should be placed alongside the scrub-up basin, for putting on before the surgeon scrubs up.

4. *Sterilisers* The small autoclave must be housed on a permanent shelf near the water and electricity supply. It must be in line with the sluicing sink and storage cabinet so that instruments, when cleaned, can then be moved straight into the steriliser, and from there either to the next operative setting on the sterile trolley (see later) or straight back into the storage cupboards thus providing a smooth flow and progression.

5. *Sluicing sink* The sink for washing and cleaning used instruments should be:

(a) Deep in design.
(b) Have its own draining area.
(c) Because of (a) and (b) a stainless steel sink with a drainer which is easy to keep clean would be ideal. Alternatively, a sink and formica topped washable shelf might be adequate.

(d) It should be situated next to the instrument storage cabinet so that when washed, cleaned and dried, the instrument setting can be checked as being complete and then be transferred either to the storage area or to be sterilised.

6. *Instrument storage cupboards* Correct instrument storage is essential in a well-run theatre set-up.

A glass plated custom-made storage cupboard is not essential as long as the principles that follow are remembered.

(a) Instruments must be kept clean and dust-free so storage must be in a cupboard or drawer of a chest which can be closed — not on an open shelf.
(b) The storage space must be able to be cleaned easily.
(c) Instruments must have their own individual, or group space, whether, for example, it be on one hook or runner to hold five artery forceps, or a single hook for scissors, etc. This means that at a glance the surgeon or assistant can tell if all the instruments are present and stored, and that one is not on its way to the garbage bin with disposable towels, etc.
(d) If possible, all the instruments used as a general basic set should be stored together and any special instruments stored separately. This makes it easier for anyone with less experience to put the correct instruments into the autoclave and not leave out anything vital when setting up for an operation.
(e) Sometimes, to facilitate storage, it helps to label the specific slots with Dymo tape or other such products.
(f) A total check list of all instruments kept in the cupboard should be available for reference and a typed list stuck to the cupboard in some visible spot is adequate.

7. *Disposable sutures and ligatures* Each surgeon will have his own preference of the size and shape of needles and the variety of ligatures, both absorbable and non-absorbable, which he will favour.

It is a good practice not to have too great a variety, yet the surgeon must be able to vary the material according to the type and size of the operation being carried out.

The sutures and needles, individually sterile packed, come in containers. Whichever firm is selected as being the one favoured by the individual surgeon, there is a rack available to hold these containers in a neat and orderly way, with their markings clearly displayed.

This rack should rest on its own shelf on the wall from which it can be removed for cleaning or, alternatively, the rack itself should be fastened to the wall as a fixture.

It should not rest on one of the working surfaces, taking up valuable room and making it more difficult to clean properly those working surfaces.

The rack should be positioned on the wall near the trolley set-up area (see below).

8. *Knife blades* Out of a variety of blades that are available perhaps a choice of three different shapes and sizes will be stocked.

   These blades come in sterile foil wraps and are contained in packets which usually have a self-feed system coming out of the bottom allowing one blade at a time in its packet, to be removed. These boxes of blades are, once again, storable on a wire frame provided by the makers. This should be a fixture alongside the sutures, fastened to the wall near the laying-up area.

9. *Gloves* Packets of the correct size of sterile pre-packed gloves in a dispenser for easy access, should be positioned near the flat surface alongside the scrub-up sink.

10. *Syringes and needles* A deliverer for sterile pre-packed 20 ml, 10 ml, 5 ml and 2 ml syringes, should be fastened to the wall alongside the suture rack and, under this, containers with a variety of different-sized needles both for drawing-up and also for fine use for infiltrating, should be available.

11. *Pathology bottles* A variety of containers, appropriately labelled for different pathological specimens, should be available, but not necessarily openly on a wall. They can be in a drawer or on a separate shelf. It is important to ensure that the stock of containers, along with request forms, is always maintained. Containers are needed for:

(a) Clotted or unclotted blood for haematological or serological examination.

(b) Histological examination with appropriate bottles containing formal saline preservative to take any operative specimens which need histological examination.

(c) Specific containers for smears, etc.

A very good place to keep these pathology requisites is in the drawer of the trolley with bandages, etc. (See later.)

12. *Laying-up area* Instruments for the operation will be on a sterile drape on a trolley alongside the surgeon and patient while the operation is proceeding.

If possible it is a very good idea to incorporate this trolley into the design of the theatre.

This means that the trolley fits into, and is stored in its place in a gap between two working surfaces on the side wall of the theatre. This facilitates storage of the trolley and, if it is designed correctly, it should be sited in a position of natural progression, following the working surface from alongside the steriliser unit. Instruments can be transferred easily, straight from the steriliser onto the trolley which has a sterile disposable towel on its surface. From there the trolley can be moved to the patient without further handling the instruments.

Thus, the laying-up area and the operating trolley are, in fact, one and the same thing.

(a) *The trolley* The trolley can be one of a variety of sizes and designs, the final choice being up to the surgeon and it is obviously influenced by that which fits into his theatre design.

Most trollies have one or two drawers under the top surface and a shelf lower down. The drawers are useful for storing bandages, dressings, plasters and wound sprays — all things needed at the end of the operation. Usually, during an operation, it is difficult for an assistant to open the drawer with the sterile instruments and drapes on the top which overlap the edge, without contaminating the whole field.

Also in these drawers can be stored pathology forms and bottles, as long as some retaining mechanism is used to ensure that the bottles, which contain the formal saline to preserve tissue for subsequent histological examination, are held upright; despite every care formal saline will leak if they fall over.

(b) *Drugs and lotions* These are again best kept in a separate, lockable cupboard.

Drugs are:

(i) Local anaesthetic agents in multidose bottles
Lignocaine 0.5%, 1%, 2%.
Lignocaine with Adrenaline 1:200.000, 0.5%, 1%.
Bupivacaine 0.25%, 0.5%.
Prilocaine 0.5%.

(ii) A small quantity of sedatives
Temazepam, Tabs. 10 mgm.
Diazepam, Tabs. 5 mgm.
Diazepam (Diazemuls) for I.V. use, ampoules of 10 mgm.

(iii) Injection of Chlorpheniramine maleate (Piriton injection 10 mgm ampoules).
Injection of Hydrocortisone, (100 mgm).
These should be available in case of some form of sensitivity reaction or allergy.

(iv) Emergency cardiac arrest kit commercially available, e.g. the emergency drug kit of IMS — International Medication Systems (UK) Ltd., Daventry, Northamptonshire NN11 5PJ. This contains:

Sodium Bicarbonate
Lignocaine
Isoprenaline
Calcium Chloride
Atropine
Adrenaline

all in a ready to use syringe system.

The box is sealed, and after use it is restocked and sealed again.

Lotions comprise the skin preparations:

(i) Hibitaine in Spirit.

(ii) Savlon — 1 in 100 — for cleansing.

Both these can be kept in 200 ml, screw-top jars to be poured by the assistant into the porringer on the trolley when required and are best kept in the drug cupboard to avoid, once again, having bottles lying around on open-top working surfaces.

13. *Disposable items* In any situation such as this, the disposable items at the end of any surgical procedure can be roughly grouped into two headings.

(a) Soft ware, i.e. soiled swabs, paper towels, drapes, etc., all of which can be disposed of by incineration, and can go into any one of many designs of disposable waste containers, usually with a liner bag of one sort or another, which can then be removed, sealed and discarded.

(b) Sharps, i.e. needles, empty glass ampules, used knife blades, syringes, etc. All of these should be put into a separate sharps' disposal box, which should be clearly marked, so that accidents do not happen with handling these disposables by them becoming inadvertently mixed with the other group.

14. *Pre-packed storage* Pre-packed sterile units will be used quite extensively. These will range from bundles of swabs to sterile drapes and complete dressing units as the complete facilities for cleaning, laundering, sterilising and autoclaving dressings and towels is too intensive.

These units, which will be discussed later, must be stored in a dry, warm area, preferably in a cupboard where they are immediately available. Each individual type of prepacked system should be stored in separate areas which are clearly marked. This will make for ease and accuracy, especially if the laying-up for an operation is being carried out by an inexperienced assistant.

These items should be protected from damage to the outer packaging which would render the whole internal packaging no longer sterile.

15. *Design and movement* When designing and positioning all the previously discussed parts of a theatre, the flow and movement of the surgeon and the flow and movement of the instruments should be considered if one has the facility to choose. (See Figure 2.2.)

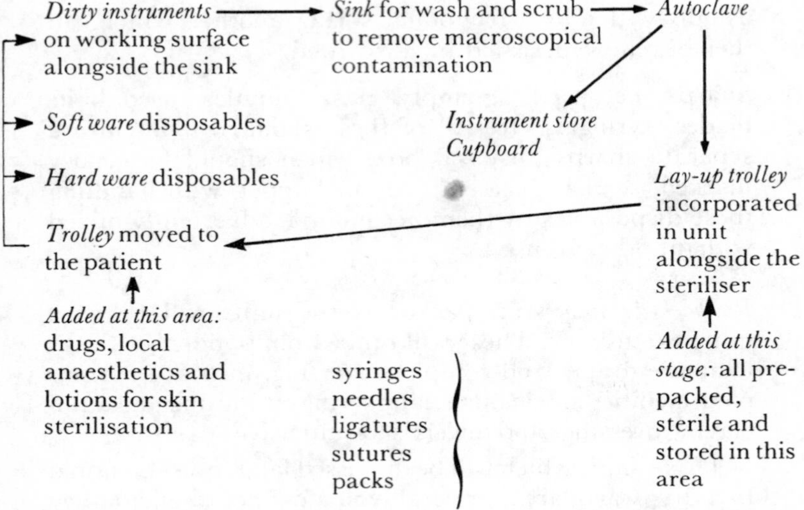

Figure 2.2 Flow and movement in the theatre

CHAPTER 3

Consultation, Note-taking and Documentation

Consultation

When the patient first presents with whatever problem is going to need surgery he is quite likely to be nervous and apprehensive.

After taking the history and carrying out the examination, the diagnosis of one of the specific conditions described later will be made and surgery proposed to the patient.

In a great number of cases if the lesion is a lump or bump the underlying fear of the patient is that a cancer has developed. It is important that in those cases where there is no possibility of this being the case, the patient should be told immediately that it is not a cancer nor is it a pre-malignant condition. The relief that this brings about is often quite profound.

The doctor should explain the condition in as much detail as he thinks necessary, that the operation can be performed by himself in one of his operating sessions and that it will be done under local anaesthetic or, alternatively, that a referral to the local hospital out patients can be arranged.

At this stage special note should be taken of the general medical state of, the patient regarding any unassociated conditions which might contraindicate the use of drugs that might be needed for the operation. Also, a detailed list must be made of all drugs and dosages that the patient is taking at that moment. All these facts must not only be recorded in the notes but also on the 'Summary Card for Surgery' — see under 'Documentation'.

This is essential as further drugs will be needed and their compatability with or antagonism to present medication must be established as, indeed, it must be known if there is any contraindication to their use due to concomittant, unassociated disease.

The patient should be questioned directly as to any known sensitivities or allergies and in particular:

1. Drugs.
2. Antibiotics and, if allergic, has this occurred with systemic or topical use?
3. Strapping or dressings which, in the past, have caused local skin sensitivity reaction and which might be used post-operatively inadvertently.
4. Skin sterilising agents such as iodine or hibitaine or their carriers, such as alcohol, which once again might have caused a previous skin sensitivity reaction.

If any sensitivity is found it should be noted on the Doctor's Operation Summary Card. It is also good practice to record any sensitivities in red ink on the front of the patient's folder and on the bottom of the Surgical Consent Form. All these documents should be available and visible pre-operatively. Some very uncomfortable, often distressing, and even dangerous sensitivity reaction can then be avoided.

It is very important at the initial consultation to gain the confidence of the patient and to allay his worries, as a relaxed patient is infinitely easier to operate upon than one tensed up and apprehensive.

Only in exceptional cases should a patient be rushed immediately from the consultation into the operating suite and the surgeon try to deal with a problem there and then — unless, of course, it is an actual emergency.

It is much better to demonstrate that the whole thing is a perfectly straightforward, routine procedure which is well organised and runs smoothly and efficiently. Because the system is so good, confidence radiates from it to the patient who becomes relaxed and confident in his turn and, in so doing, half the battle is won.

Time must be spent on explaining to the patient exactly what is going to happen and the way that it is organised.

A superficial explanation of the operation should be given, and this can be done as the documentation (see later) is being completed so that the explanation proceeds regularly step by step with the documentation and any questions can be asked and answered at that time. Indeed, it is good practice to encourage a reticent patient to ask questions rather than hold back and worry.

Note keeping

The system for keeping patients' records of past history, examination, special investigations, diagnoses and treatment, and the widespread documentation associated with this, varies in different practices with each doctor having his own personal preference and ideas.

Some keep their notes loosely in folders, some on cards, some loose in envelopes. Some doctors make extensive notes, some very brief, and all have their own personal system, developed and improved with time, which works best for them and should not be altered.

However, for any surgery, there is specific documentation which must be carried out and this is best done at the original consultation. There is also documentation which is not essential but which helps both doctor and the patient and which will be suggested for consideration.

Documentation

1. Patient reminder form.
2. Consent for operation form.
(a) Adult patient.
(b) Parent or guardian for a minor.
(c) Male sterilisation form.
3. Summary card for notes.

Patient reminder form

The patient may be worried or apprehensive when seen at the original consultation and some of the details and explanations given to him may not be remembered.

It is very helpful to the patient if a typed sheet with a summary of these instructions can be provided which he can then take home with him after the initial consultation.

This sheet is then available for the patient to refer back to as necessary and thus avoid confusion and subsequent telephone calls, enquiries and perhaps inevitable postponement of a planned procedure.

Patient reminder form

Surgery Address ....

Patient's Name ....

Patient's Address ....

.... Tel. No. ....

The operation which, Dr. .... advised you to have carried out by him, will be done at the surgery, at the above address, on .... at ....

This will be carried out under local anaesthetic which means that the area will be anaesthetised but you yourself will be fully awake.

You may be given a sedative which should be taken at .... on .... and you should be accompanied and brought to the surgery one hour later at .... on ....

On the same day as the operation you may have a light meal three hours before you are due to report to the surgery, but after that meal you should have only fluids by mouth as desired. These fluids may include tea, coffee or milk drinks, but no alcohol in any form.

The area which needs to be shaved will have been outlined for you by the doctor and you should make arrangements to have that area shaved and afterwards well washed, the evening before the surgery.

Due to the sedation you will be unable to drive your car either to or from the surgery and therefore it is advisable to have a friend accompany you to the surgery and also to make arrangements for a companion to escort you home after the procedure.

If, for any reason, you are unable to keep this appointment please notify the surgery immediately so that arrangements can be made for someone else to make use of the operating time you have vacated.

An appointment has been arranged for you to return to the surgery on .... at .... for the doctor to check the operation and remove any stitches which have been inserted.

This certainly is recommended to facilitate the orderly, well-organised running of the operation session.

A suggested format for this explanation reminder is as follows, although obviously it can be modified by the doctor concerned to suit his own surgery arrangements. Once a satisfactory format is arrived at it can then be cyclostyled or photostated and the patient given it fully filled in, with the exception of the follow-up appointment time which is entered after the operation is completed.

Anaesthetic and operative consent form

This form should be signed by the patient or, if a child is under age, by the legal guardian or parent.

Section 8 of The Family Law Reform Act 1969 provides that the consent to medical, surgical or dental treatment of a minor who has attained the age of 16 years shall be effective consent and that in such cases it is not necessary to obtain consent forms from the parent or guardian.

The actual format of the anaesthetic and operative consent form can vary but the one following (2a) is the one recommended by The Medical Defence Union.

Copies of this consent form should be available so that, at the first visit to the surgery when the surgical procedure is being discussed and decided upon, the forms can be signed.

It is much better medically and legally to get the form signed at that visit. If it is delayed to the actual day of the operation it will be signed by the patient who may be, at that moment, under sedation. This just might present complications in the future that could well be avoided.

As in all surgical procedures, the form should be filled in legibly and the precise diagnosis and proposed operative treatment written in full. This acts as a double check if necessary at the time of operation.

Also, it is a very good principle and practice as far as the completion of the forms is concerned, that no abbreviations should be used. In particular, the side of the operation should be written in full as 'left' or 'right' and not as 'L' or 'R' which might be mistaken or misread at a later date.

If any procedure is going to be carried out on a digit, that digit must be described and not just numbered, and thus a hand is not only documented as to the side but also whether it is the thumb, index finger, middle finger, ring finger or little finger which is to be operated upon.

Also, it must be documented in the notes whether it is the dorsal or palmar surface and, if possible, the precise location related to interphalangeal or metocarpo-phalangeal or metatarso-phalangeal joints.

Consent by Patient

Surgery Address ....

....

I, ... of ....

....

hereby consent to undergo the operation of ....

....

the nature and purpose of which have been explained to me by Dr./Mr. ....

I also consent to such further or alternative operative measures as may be found to be necessary during the course of the operation and to the administration of a local anaesthetic for any of these purposes.

Date .... (Signed) ....
(Patient)

I confirm that I have explained to the patient the nature and purpose of this operation.

Date .... (Signed) ....
(Medical Practitioner)

Consent by Parent or Guardian

Surgery Address ....

....

Patient's Name ....

I, ... of ....

....

the parent/guardian of the above-named, hereby consent to the submission of my child to the operation of

....

the nature and purpose of which has been explained to me by Dr./Mr. ....

I also consent to such further or alternative operative measures as may be found to be necessary during the course of the operation and to the administration of a local anaesthetic for any of these purposes.

Date .... (Signed) ....
(Parent/Guardian)

I confirm that I have explained to the child's parent/guardian the nature and purpose of this operation.

Date .... (Signed) ....
(Medical Practitioner)

A cyst, a ganglion or other lesion which is to be excised and which when seen originally was obvious and standing out well, may subsequently, when the patient arrives for surgery, be very much smaller or have altered in some other way. In these circumstances, even though the patient is not under general anaesthetic, it is vitally important to have the documentation accurate and legible.

Consent to male sterilisation — married man

This form, as detailed below, should be signed by the patient and his wife together at the consultation at which the final decision is made to carry out the vasectomy sterilisation on the husband.

It must be signed by both parties at the same time and the form must also be completed by the surgeon at the same time, and dated. No vasectomy under any circumstances should ever be carried out without the completion of this form.

Very occasionally technical difficulties do arise with the signing of this form when a vasectomy is desired by a couple who at that present moment are not married. If the doctor is agreeable to carry out the vasectomy for the man in those circumstances, then the form must be amended to read:

I, (then unmarried name of wife-to-be), (following which she should write) 'intended wife of the above'.

Very occasionally the problem also arises of a man requesting vasectomy who has been for some time separated from but is not yet divorced from his wife. Legally there is no necessity for the man to obtain the written consent of his wife. For further discussion of these points, see under 'Operations/ Vasectomy'.

Summary Card for Surgery

To facilitate the smooth running of a minor operative session, a card with the following details should be filled in at the initial consultation and be available with the notes at the operating session.

A card such as this with all the essentials summarised obviates the necessity to be searching through notes to check on drugs or sensitivities or other medical conditions before the operation begins.

All the documentation is seen to be completed and if there is any doubt in the surgeon's mind he can then search the notes for more precise information about that particular point. Some practitioners have found this helpful whereas others consider it

Consent for primary sterilisation

Surgery Address ....

....

I, ... of ....

....

hereby consent to undergo the operation of vasectomy, the nature of which has been explained to me by Dr./Mr.

....

I have been told that the object of the operation is to render me sterile and incapable of parenthood. I understand that the effect of the operation is not guaranteed due to the possibility that reversal may occur naturally in the future thus leading to renewed fertility.
I consent to the administration of a local or other anaesthetic.

Date .... (Signed) ....
(Patient)

Agreement by Spouse

I .... the wife of the abovenamed, being over twenty-one years hereby agree to the operation of vasectomy being carried out on my husband, the nature and effect of which has been explained to my by Dr./Mr. .... I have read and understand the whole of this form and it has been signed by my husband in my presence.

Date .... (Signed) ....
(Spouse)

I confirm that I have explained the nature and effect of this operation to the patient and his spouse.

Date .... (Signed) ....
(Medical Practitioner)

to be an over-sophistication. However, two points should be made.

1. It does contain all the details of the operation on one sheet which can be stored in the notes and which can be referred back to if further surgery is needed at a later date.
2. If one doctor in the practice is carrying out the surgery for other partners in his practice whose patients he does not know as well as his own, a summary such as this can save a lot of worry and difficulty if it is filled in by the patient's own doctor.

Summary Card for Surgery

The card suggested has a format as follows:

Name of Patient ....

Surgical Procedure ....

Date ....

Present drug medication ....

....

....

Known sensitivities ....

....

....

Documentation

Surgical & Anaesthetic Consent signed ....

....

Primary Sterilisation Consent signed ....

....

....

Anaesthetic used ....

Surgical Procedure Notes ....

....

....

CHAPTER 4

Instruments

Selection

The selection and choice of any instrument is a very personal matter. The general type of category of instrument is predetermined in any operation and thus one needs a knife or scissors to cut, or artery forceps or haemostats to control bleeding, etc.

Having decided on the main groups of instruments needed, there are a great number of variations on the same theme. The field is therefore narrowed down for consideration.

Knife

The days of having the integral one-piece scalpel which was sharpened and honed with great care and affection have now passed and the knife is now usually a two-part instrument.

The first part is the handle which comes in varying lengths and holds one of two blade sizes, each particular size taking a selection of blades. These blades vary in shape and size, and each has its own advantages. In the final analysis the choice rests with the individual surgeon as to which feels right to him.

The scalpel handle has to be sterilised, whereas the blades, which come prepacked in sterile packets, are used once and then discarded. The handles are designated by numbers, Number 3 being designed to take the smaller range of knife blades. Handle Number 4 is designed to take the upper range.

The design of the handle is fairly constant and certainly on any operative setting there should be one of each size.

A selection of blade shapes and sizes is illustrated (Figure 4.1). As it is impractical to keep a full range of different sizes and shapes, the initial choice of which one is thought to be most suitable is important, and attention should be directed to the combination of shapes of blades of the two sizes as well as to their individual merits.

Figure 4.1 Selection of blade shapes and sizes

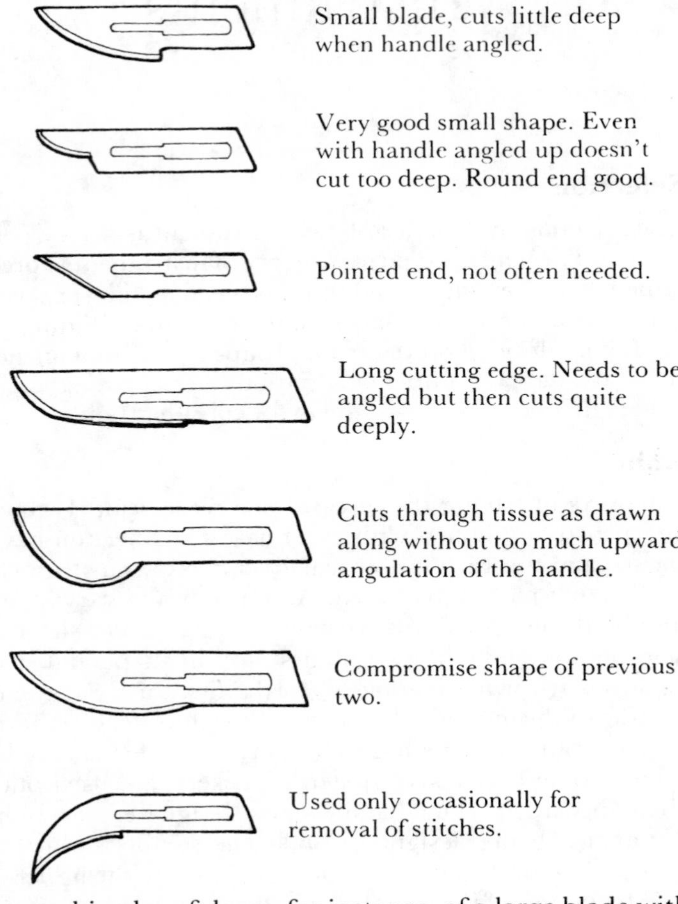

The combined usefulness, for instance, of a large blade with a pointed tip would perhaps compliment one of the smaller blades with a rounded end for fine dissection or, alternatively, the rounded end of a large blade might well be preferred and this combined with the pointed end of the finer blade.

In later chapters discussing the technique of the surgery, the availability of both sizes of blades will once again become obvious.

Scissors

Scissors are precision tools. The cutting power at the tip of a pair of scissors depends upon the shearing effect of one accurately ground blade against another and therefore their accuracy is destroyed by any misuse which:

(a) Springs or distorts one of the blades so that they oppose accurately only near the joint and not at the tip.

(b) Loosens the joint, whether it be a screw joint or a box joint which, in order to keep the blades opposed, necessitates the blades being pulled together with the fingers whilst cutting.

(c) Loses the accuracy of the honing of the edges due to rusting or cutting the wrong material with the wrong instrument.

There should, therefore, be on the operating set the following:

1. A pair of heavy, straight, flat-nosed scissors for cutting dressings, sutures or other heavy work.
2. Fine, curved, blunt-nosed scissors for most fine dissecting work.
3. Straight, fine, sharp-pointed scissors for fine dissection work or removal of fine stitches.

As the surgery envisaged is relatively superficial, all the scissors should be within the range of 15 cms to 20 cms long.

1. ***Dressing scissors*** The choice of this type of scissor is not very wide as it is a fairly standard instrument. (Figure 4.2)

Figure 4.2 Dressing scissors

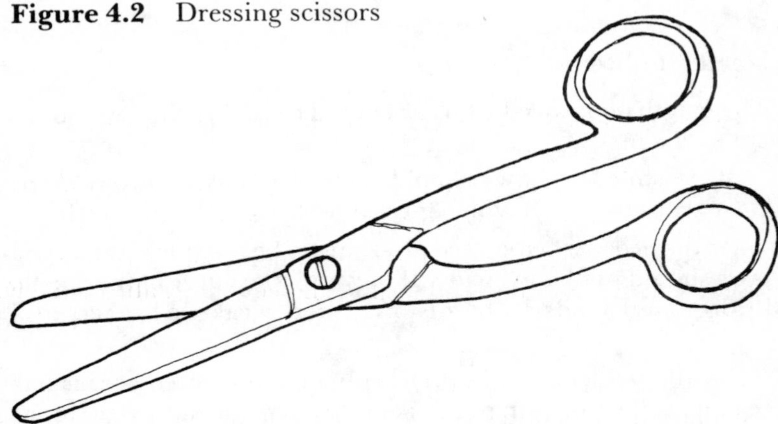

2. ***Fine-curved scissors*** Most sets of scissors are screw-jointed and not box-jointed and variation is due to:
(a) The length of the blade from the joint to the tip.
(b) The degree of curvature of the blade which is curved on the flat.
(c) The relative blunting of the tip.

A popular, well-used and tried design is the Mayo Scissors which seem to combine a good combination of all these points. (Figure 4.3)

Figure 4.3 Mayo scissors

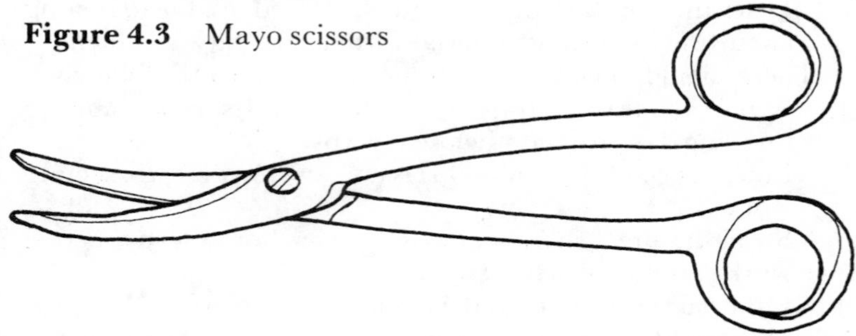

3. ***Sharp-pointed scissors, or stitch scissors*** Once again, because these are a very standard instrument, variation is not very great.

Needle holders

The length of the needle holder should be within the range of 15 cm to 20 cm.

If possible, the jaws should have a Tungsten insert or be Carbarundum-lined which gives a better grip on the needle.

As the needles being used are going to be relatively small, the jaws should not be too wide. If they are, the curve of the needle bridges and tends to be distorted and weakened when it is gripped.

Needle holders should preferably be box-jointed as this has the advantage of being less likely to snag the suture material when using the instrument to tie knots.

With the above criterion the variety of needle holders can be classified as follows:

Those shaped rather similarly to a straight artery forcep or haemostat, the main difference being that the distance between the tip of the needle holder and the joint is very much shorter than the distance in the haemostat because in the needle-holder a small length gives a great deal more holding power due to the leverage.

This type of needle holder has many variations but can be subdivided into:

(a) Those which close and clip, thus securing the needle without further pressure.

(b) Those that need a constant pressure to hold the needle in the jaws.

The first category (a) is the most popular overall, although the design of this type of instrument once again does vary and two such designs are illustrated.

Debakey needle holder This is a simple box-jointed light-weight needle holder with Tungsten Carbide-faced jaws which clips like a straight artery forcep, the whole instrument being in the one plane. (Figure 4.4)

Figure 4.4 Debakey needle holder

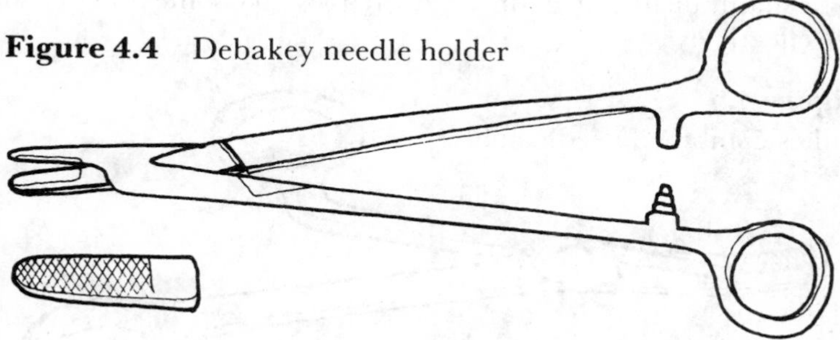

Kilner needle holder This, as seen in the illustration (Figure 4.5), closes like an artery forcep, also has a Tungsten jaw but is off-set from the handle end. Some operators find this improves the view of the needle as it moves it a little bit away from any obscuring by the fingers.

The second category (b) contains those that need constant pressure to hold the needle in place.

Figure 4.5 Kilner needle holder

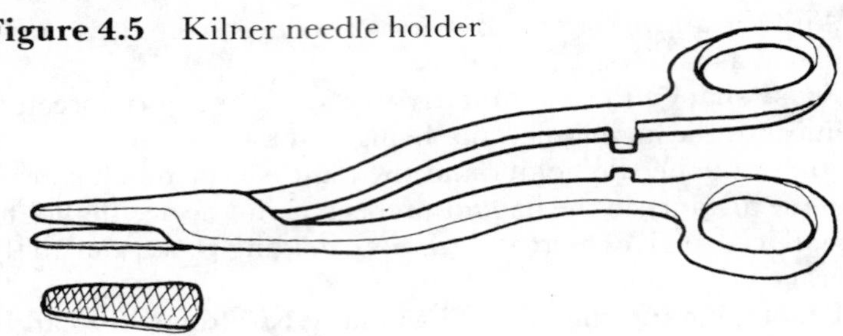

Gillies combined needle holder This is the most popular design. The combined needle holder and scissors is illustrated (Figure 4.6). The advantage of this instrument is that the thumb and finger hole are offset and angled which makes prolonged use that bit more comfortable. In particular, when a surgeon is likely to be working with limited assistance, the Gillies combined needle holder, can be used as a needle holder to put in the stitch, as an instrument to help to tie the knot, and to cut the suture material without having to change to a second instrument, i.e. a pair of scissors. This has a great deal to offer.

This is a very good instrument but as constant pressure has to be maintained to grip the needle it does take some practice to use effectively.

Figure 4.6
Gillies combined needle holder

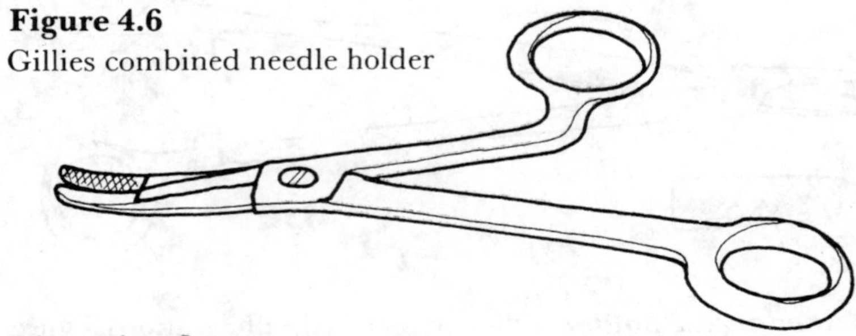

Dissecting forceps

A dissecting forcep is an instrument designed to grip tissue firmly so that dissection may be carried out in that particular area without the tissue being damaged.

When in the resting position a dissecting forcep lies with its tips open and when used for gripping tissue it has to be closed against the spring effect of the proximal end. If this forcep is to be used for any length of time this resistance against the finger grip must not be too great as this induces a degree of tiredness and cramp and thus loss of accuracy.

So, in selecting the instrument, the resistance offered to opposition of the blades should be assessed to be comfortable for prolonged usage.

Likewise, the handle to be gripped by the fingers should not only feel comfortable but should be designed so that it is not too smooth allowing the fingers to slip, and not too narrow so that the instrument tends to twist.

Having considered these points, when deciding upon the best handle of the dissecting forceps the varieties can further be classified depending on the type and format of the gripping end or jaws.

As well as holding tissue which varies between deep, soft tissue and firmer skin, the forcep must be designed to grip a curved needle firmly and accurately. This is so that when tissue or skin is being stitched with a curved needle held in a needle holder, the dissecting forcep can hold the needle firmly in position while the needle holder is removed from the shank of the needle and replaced on that part of the needle which has traversed the tissue being sutured.

Thus, the variety of dissecting forceps are many and excluding the type of grip and the strength of opposition can be, perhaps, classified as follows:

(a) The end of the jaw can be wide or narrow.

(b) The end of the jaw can be either plain or interlocking at its tip with one or more teeth, the teeth of one blade interlocking with the gaps between the teeth of the other blade.

Tooth forceps tend to grip skin and deep tissue very well, but because of their format they can also be very traumatic, causing damage to the tissue held. If that tissue is skin, the damage can be reflected in puncture marks which subsequently cause added unsightly scarring.

Plain forceps, without teeth, rely on their gripping power by pressure so, once again, if used harshly they damage the tissue by crushing rather than by the impaling which is caused by the teeth of the toothed forcep.

(c) The gripping surface of the forcep can have (i) transverse grooves, (ii) longitudinal grooves, (iii) a hatched surface.

Of these many variations the following points should be considered before deciding which forceps should be acquired for the operating set.

The surface with gripping grooves on some forceps is built up on a shoulder so that the surfaces are parallel on opposition, whereas in the majority of the forceps the surface just coincides at its tip when closed and there is a slight gap proximal to it (see Figure 4.7) which closes and approximates only with further pressure.

Figure 4.7 Type of gripping surface on the majority of forceps

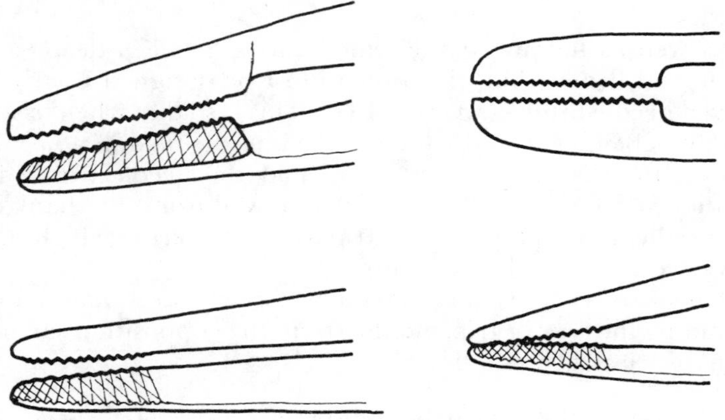

As the forcep has to grip a needle as well as tissue, in general the ones with the transverse grooves do not afford such a good grip. The needle tends to slip between the grooves and, therefore, for this sort of operative set these should not be used if one instrument for universal use is desired.

The hatched grip, overall, is very much better and affords the best performance. (Figure 4.8.)

Although it looks a little bulky and inelegant, an ideal dissecting forcep which grips without crushing and also grips a needle well, at whichever angle the needle is presented, is the Mayo or Russian Forcep (Figure 4.9). The wide end spreads

Figure 4.8
Hatched gripping surface

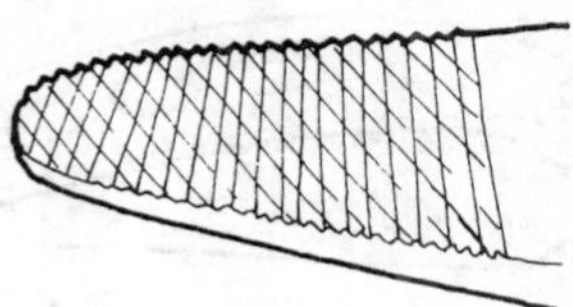

out the tension which tends to mitigate the crushing effect. The grooves are not deep enough to cause tissue damage and they are radially placed which facilitates a firm grip on both tissue and needle; there are no teeth to impale and damage tissue. Overall, this instrument is considered to be very good but, in view of the width of its end and the small incisions, its use is limited. Therefore, there should also be a pair of medium width, non-tooth forceps with longitudinal or hatched grooves, and a pair of fine-toothed dissecting forceps, making three types in all.

Toothed forceps, which fulfil most of the design features already suggested, include Jean Dissecting Forceps (Figure 4.10) which, although very comfortable to use, with a good grip and parallel-closing jaws, do have the disadvantage of transverse grooves. Alternatively, Ramsay Dissecting Forceps have parallel opposing jaws with a hatched surface and a very good gripping handle. (Figure 4.11.)

The non-toothed forceps are mainly designed with transverse grooves as these are not so often used to grip a needle, and their variation is usually in the design of the handle rather than the jaws of the instrument.

Figure 4.9
Mayo or Russian forcep

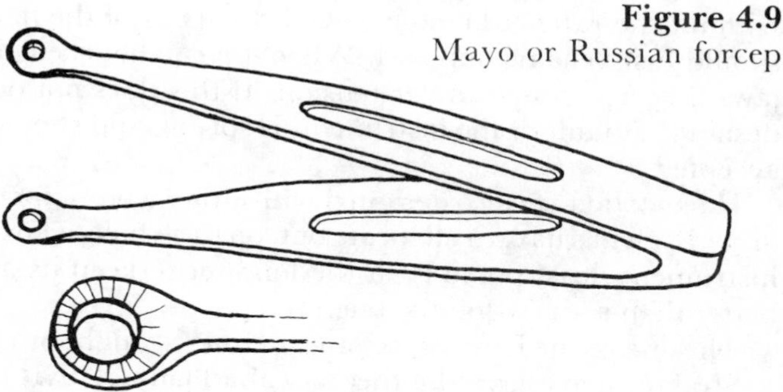

Figure 4.10
. Jean dissecting forcep

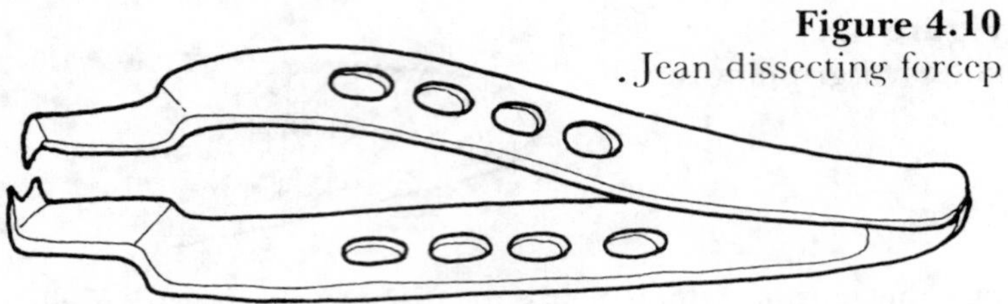

Figure 4.11 Ramsay dissecting forcep

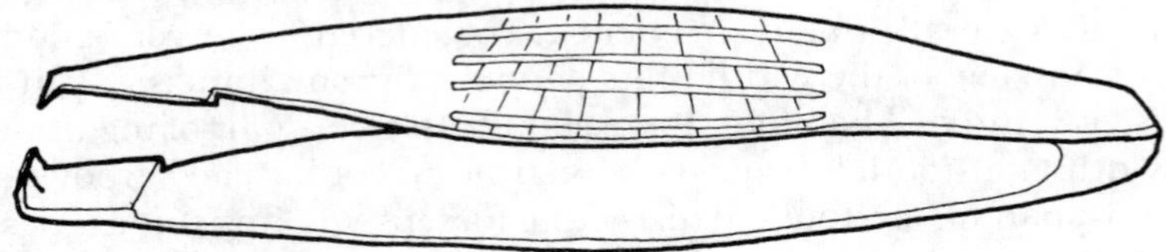

Artery forceps or haemostats

To arrest bleeding by closing a haemostat on the bleeding point, the end of the instrument must be fine and close accurately. Having been closed, the clip at the handle which keeps it so, does its job and does not spring open.

The handle end of haemostats are fairly constant in design, having an equal-sized thumb and finger hole at the same level from the joint. The different handle designs vary only in the number of ratchets which are present to hold the instrument closed.

When gently opposed at the handle end up to the ratchet, without the ratchet being engaged, the jaws of the haemostat should just become opposed. When the ratchet is engaged the jaws are then closed under tension. If this does not occur the design is at fault or the instrument is sprung and should not be accepted.

Haemostats are also designed with either a box joint or screw joint. Each has its own advocate but, on the whole, a box-jointed instrument does, possibly in the long term, keep its accuracy better than a screw-jointed one.

The end of the haemostat can be either straight or curved.

Straight ends have the theoretical advantage that they can

be more easily directed onto a bleeding point as they are in direct line with the instrument, rather than one that is curved away from that line.

A curved end to the haemostat has the advantage that when the vessel is secured and has to be ligated, the ligature is more easily and safely applied. This is because, due to its shape, the point of the instrument can be lifted a little and the ligature slipped over it and around the underlying vessel more easily than the straight forcep.

Once again it is a matter of personal choice, but on balance it is suggested that for the form of surgery that is envisaged, the curved haemostat would be more suitable.

The end of the instrument, although being fine, must not be pointed or sharp as this can cause additional tissue damage; a fine blunt-nose end should be aimed for. Also, the ends must oppose accurately because if one blade protrudes this snags vessels and creates further bleeding. So, when buying each instrument it should be held up to the light to check that there is no overlap at the tip.

The delicacy of the forcep ranges from a fine Halstead Mosquito Artery Forcep up to a quite heavy Spencer Wells Forcep and one should be chosen somewhere in the intervening range or, alternatively, a group of the two different types is ideal.

The grooves on the jaws of the forceps are very important and although most designs have transverse grooves, there are some, such as the Grey Turner Artery Forcep, which have a combination of hatched and longitudinal grooves which grip very well. (Figure 4.12.)

Figure 4.12 Grey Turner artery forcep

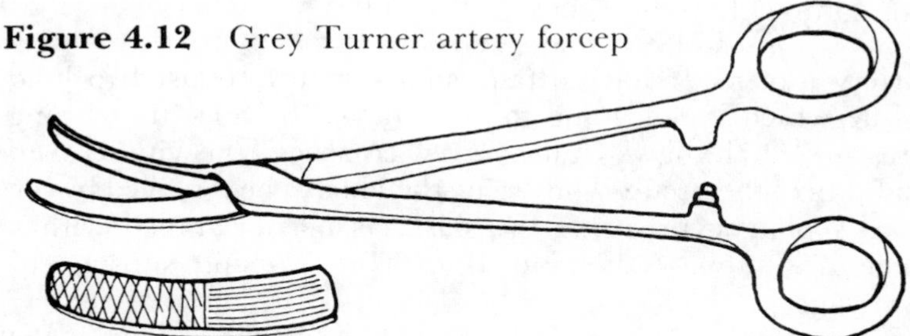

Whichever groove pattern is decided upon it is very important that the pattern is continued all the way up the blade of the forcep to the joint and is not grooved only for a short way up from the tip. With such an instrument if, in an emergency, a large bite of tissue has to be taken to control haemostasis, that part of the instrument near the joint will not grip and will slip.

Heavy artery forceps Sometimes it is necessary to grip a large bite of tissue, such as a nail when removing it, and one should not under any circumstances use the normal artery forceps for this procedure as it can cause the jaws to spring and to lose their accuracy. Therefore, in the proposed surgical set, two heavy artery forceps should also be included for this sort of work. These can be either straight or curved and, as they have to grip a large bulk of tissue, they should be one design with a tooth at the end of the jaws to lock it into place when closed. The forceps with this design feature are either Ochsner Artery Forceps or Kocher Artery Forceps.

These forceps can also be used to hold dissected dabs and two are a useful addition to the set (Figure 4.13).

Figure 4.13 Design of Ochsner artery forcep and Kocher artery forcep

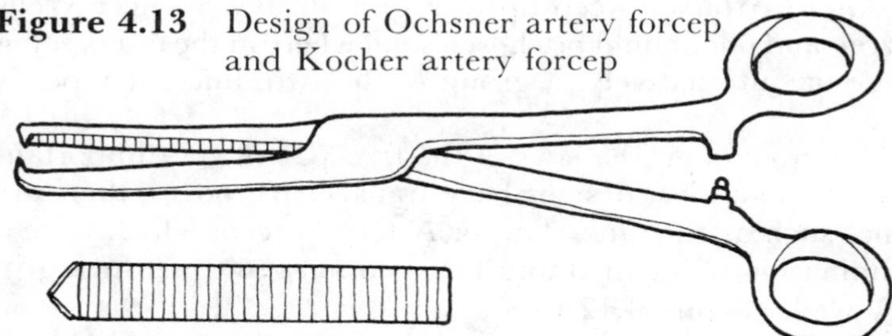

Tissue forceps

Artery forceps or haemostats, should never be used to hold tissue which is not going to be removed because the closing pressure of the jaws destroys, by crushing, the vitality and viability of the tissue. This tissue then has to be removed by the body's phagocytes or, if the skin has been clamped with a haemostat, this disaster leads to skin loss and subsequent scarring.

Tissue forceps are so designed that when the ratchet at the

handle end is closed and locked, the blades are still not opposed but remain open by approximately 2 mm, with the aim of minimising damage to the tissue being held.

It must be said, however, that this theory does not always hold good and, if tissue forceps are used on the skin or deep tissue without due care, there is usually some damage, with resultant scarring left in the future. As a matter of technique it is infinitely preferable to use skin hooks on the skin. Skin hooks are more delicate and precise. They give minimal tissue damage, and should be used rather than tissue forceps on the skin (see overleaf).

If fat or deep tissue is needed to be held, then the tissue forceps should be used. The design of the tissue forceps is, at the handle end, the same as an artery forcep, with the thumb and finger holes being at the same level and there being a ratchet which closes with a various number of steps.

When the tissue forcep is closed and the ratchet is gently opposed but not engaged, the jaws of the instrument should be fairly widely open. When the ratchet is engaged on its first step they should remain separate and not close completely. There should be a gap of at least 2 mm even when the ratchet is fully closed.

The joint of the instrument can, once again, be screw-jointed or box-jointed, the latter being preferable.

Figure 4.14 Jaw designs

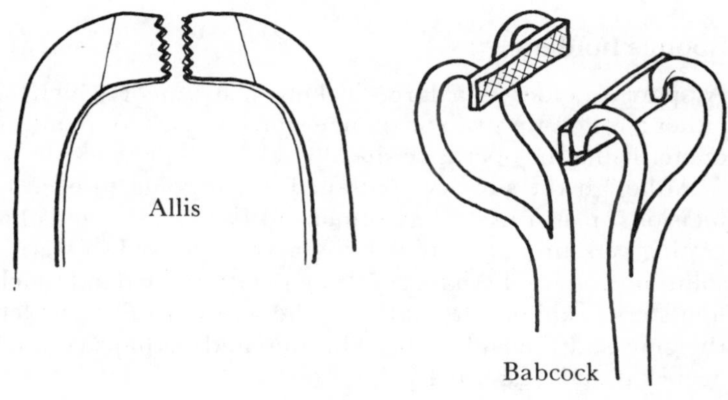

The length of the instrument should, again, be in the 15 cm to 20 cm range as any deeper dissection is not envisaged.

The design of the end of the instrument varies, from the fine teeth of the Allis to the bar-type blade of the Babcock.

As the Babcock Tissue Forcep, due to the curved design of its blade, can be used as a holding forcep in operations such as vasectomy, it is suggested that this design should be the one selected.

(See illustration for jaw designs, Figure 4.14.)

Skin hooks

These are finely tempered, sharp-pointed yet delicate, curved hooks, which are used to retract or, alternatively, tension skin.

By being hooked in the under-surface of the skin, scarring is reduced to a minimum. They are a very useful adjunct for retraction and sometimes also a help when suturing skin. By being applied at each end of the incision the tension on them approximates the skin edges accurately for the stitches to be applied.

They are much less traumatic than tissue forceps and very useful. A good design is that of Gillies Small Size. (Figure 4.15.)

Figure 4.15 Gillies small size skin hook

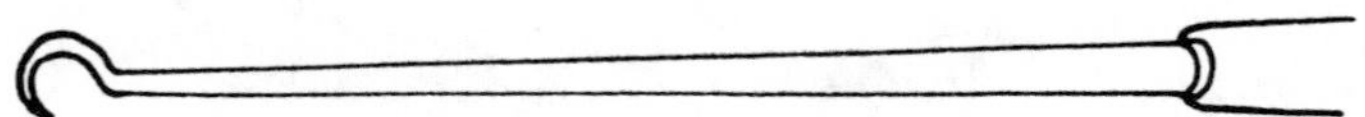

Sponge holders

A sponge holder is a large locking instrument which holds either a rolled-up swab or sponge which is used for painting up or sterilising the operative site.

Although the surgery envisaged is not going to need large incisions, it is a useful instrument to have as it avoids hands getting contaminated by holding a swab soaked in sterilising solution close to the skin, resulting in either the hand touching non-sterile skin or, alternatively, the solution still being left on the gloves at the end of the skin prep and perhaps contacting deeper tissue. (Figure 4.16.)

Figure 4.16 Sponge holder

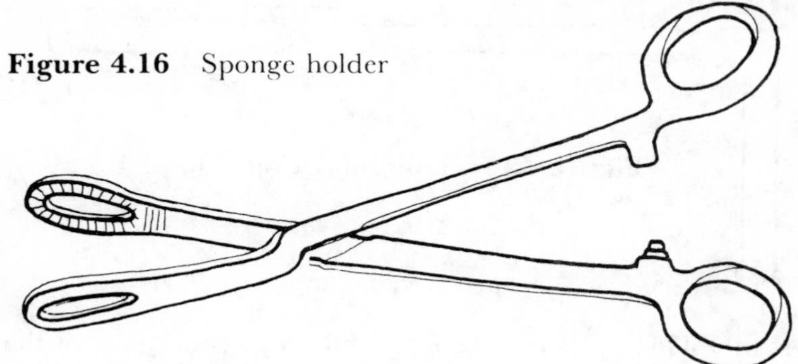

Retractors

These can be divided into: (a) those held by the hand, and (b) a self-retaining retractor.

Hand-held retractors As discussed before, skin should be retracted preferably with fine skin hooks rather than by any hand-held retractor as the skin hooks are very much less traumatic.

However, sub-cutaneous fat and deeper tissues have to be retracted with a deeper instrument to facilitate the view for any deeper dissection.

The best design of hand-held retractor is that of Langenbeck. This is a right-angled retractor, with a lip, which is rounded and as atraumatic as it is possible to design, and it has a good handle which ensures a firm, non-slip grip.

Some hand-held retractors have a blade at one end and a claw at the other but this multiple instrument is not recommended as, when holding it, the claw quite often damages the glove. As a claw, in principle, does tend to be a traumatic type of retractor, this end of the hook is not often used.

Other double-ended, right-angled retractors are also made but these have the disadvantage that the protruding end at the hand end of the instrument, tends to limit the angle at which the blade, that is retracting, be applied. Also, the design does not enable a good, easy handle to be incorporated.

Thus, the Langenbeck type of retractor with a good handle, a right-angled blade with a further right-angled tip (Figure 4.17)

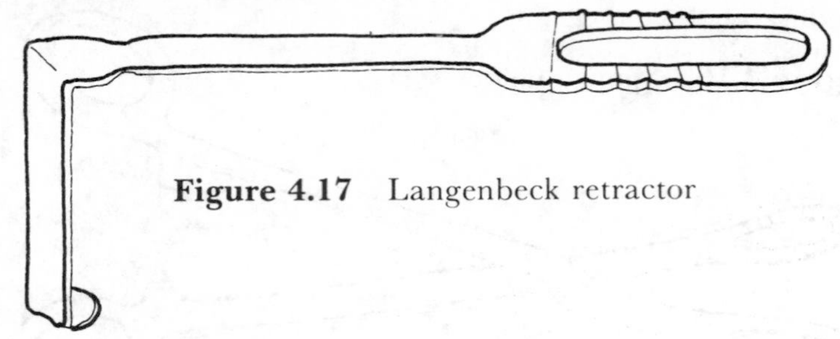

Figure 4.17 Langenbeck retractor

— the blade lip being rounded and an essential part of the retractor to help avoid it slipping out — are the features which should be incorporated in any choice of hand retractor.

Self-retaining retractors The principle of a self-retaining retractor is one of having two blades which by some expanding mechanism can widen out after being placed in the incision and, having been widened out to the required distance, are then locked.

Unfortunately, most self-retaining retractors have the blades of a claw design, rather than a softer, more atraumatic flat surface as the latter does tend to slip.

Some of the self-retaining retractor designs have blades which are removable and replaceable by a different variety of size. Others of this type of retractor do not have blades but have a clipping mechanism whereby the tissue is clipped with a pointed self-locking clip on each side, such as Jolls Retractor used in thyroidectomy. Both these aforementioned types are not ideally suited for the type of surgery that is envisaged, as both are liable to cause trauma if not used correctly, and are too big and complicated.

The locking mechanism of a self-retaining retractor can be either on the principle of an artery forcep or needle holder where there is an extensive ratchet and the closure of the handle up this ratchet opens the jaw until the necessary tension is achieved and, having done so, the jaws remain open at that level until released. Alternatively, the jaws can be opened and kept open by a screw mechanism which is tightened at the handle end and once again holds the jaws firmly apart.

The third general method is a spring mechanism at the

handle end of the instrument and it is used by closing the jaws against this resistance and then allowing them to open, being pulled open by the spring and thus the wound is retracted, not as a constant size but against this ever-present tension.

Figure 4.18 Design of Travers retractor and Mastoid retractor

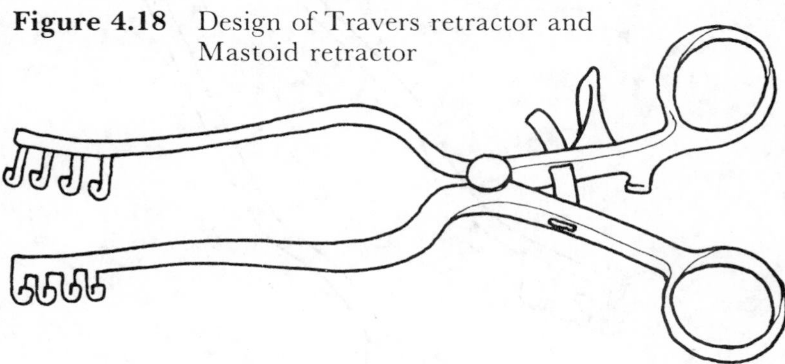

Of the three types, generally the Travers or Mastoid Retractor design (Figure 4.18) will probably have the widest use, although the spring type, called the Newton Searby Retractor, is also illustrated (Figure 4.19) but, if chosen, the spring tension must not be too great as tissue damage may result.

Extras

Any surgical set has a whole bundle of 'extras' which are personal, perhaps unusual, instruments that a particular operator has found to merit a permanent place in his set.

Some surgeons would rate some of the extras which will be discussed now as being an essential part of any setting, whereas others would use them so infrequently that they would hardly rate their inclusion.

'Jimmy' This is the name given to a James Macdonald Dissector (Figure 4.20). It is a simple instrument which is double-ended, having a blunt flat end at one end and the same type of surface but bent at the other end.

It is an invaluable instrument for dissecting out tissue planes or getting behind things one cannot see properly, etc. and is recommended as being well worthwhile including in a set.

Figure 4.19 Newton Searby retractor

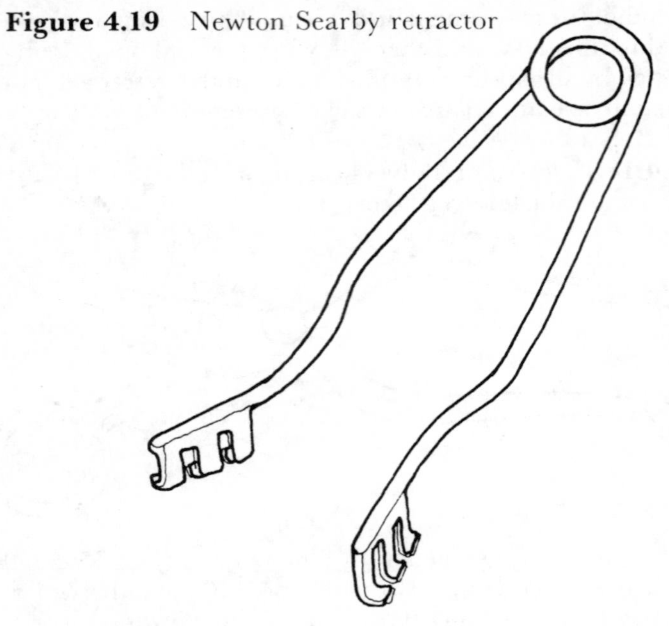

Figure 4.20 James Macdonald dissector

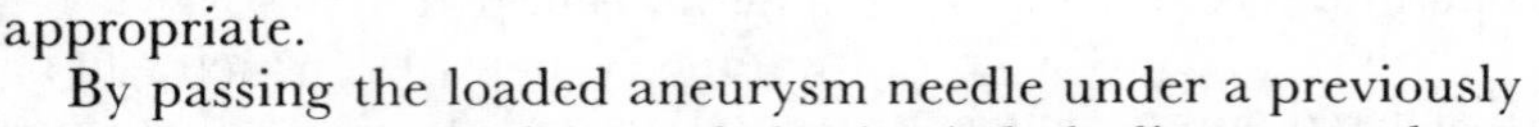

Aneurysm needles The aneurysm needle is a simple curved blunt-ended hook on a handle with a hole near the tip through which can be threaded catgut or other suture material as appropriate.

By passing the loaded aneurysm needle under a previously dissected vessel, which is needed to be tied, the ligature end can then be held and the needle withdrawn back the way it was inserted and removed along the ligature, leaving it under the vessel to be tied.

The advantage of the aneurysm needle is that if assistance is not available and it is necessary to tie a vessel, it is safer to tie it in two places using an aneurysm needle and dividing the vessel between the ties, i.e. in continuity, than it is to put on a haemostat or artery forcep in two places, divide between them and then have to tie the vessel, releasing the artery forcep as the knot is being tightened which, one-handed, can present problems to the inexperienced.

Also, the alternative is to pass a tie under the vessel by passing an artery forcep under the vessel and pulling the tie through with it. Sometimes when this manoeuvre is attempted, when the artery forcep is under the vessel and is closed to grip the tie, the anterior surface of the forcep sometimes snags on the undersurface of the vessel that is being encircled causing it to tear and bleed.

The basic design of the aneurysm needle can vary as to the direction of the hook in relation to the direction of the handle. As long as the handle offers a firm grip, which does not slip, and the end of the aneurysm needle itself is not in any way sharp or pointed, and the hole is big enough to enable the operator to thread his ligature material through it without too much frustration, then the design is one of personal preference (Figure 4.21).

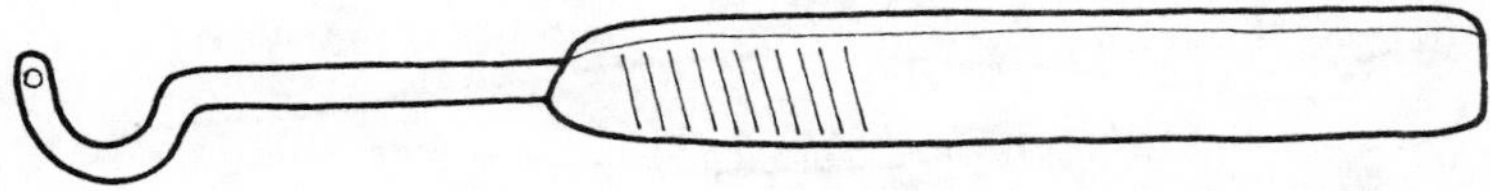

Figure 4.21 Aneurysm needle

Probes A malleable blunt-nosed probe to explore any sinous tract is a well worthwhile extra.

No probe should be so fine that there is a danger when it is used of it penetrating the wall of the tract it is traversing, making a false passage. The most useful is, therefore, a medium-thickness, blunt-ended probe which should be able to be bent if necessary to facilitate its passage.

Some probes are so designed that having a blunt end they also have the shaft proximal to that grooved. The aim and object of this is to guide the blade of a knife along the groove when the probe is actually in the tract and thus, by cutting up to the groove, the tract is laid open. As it is unlikely that this is going to be needed for the surgery contemplated, and as the actual groove means that the shaft of the probe is that much thicker, the simple ungrooved probe is the one that would be most used.

A malleable retractor This is, in essence, a flat piece of copper with rounded edges and rounded corners which can be bent to form a retractor of the surgeon's own design as required at any specific moment of difficulty. With a Langenbeck retractor already in the set, the malleable retractor is not often needed but, on the other hand, it can—on occasions—prove to be an invaluable tool and well worth the small cost needed to include it amongst the extras.

Curette or Scoop A scoop is a very useful instrument for curetting or scraping out the granulation tissue and debris from an abscess cavity wall or warts. It rather resembles a deep small spoon with a sharpened rim.

There are various designs but to cut down the number of instruments, the double-ended type of scoop with a medium-sized bowl, such as a Volkmann, is very useful and should be included (Figure 4.22).

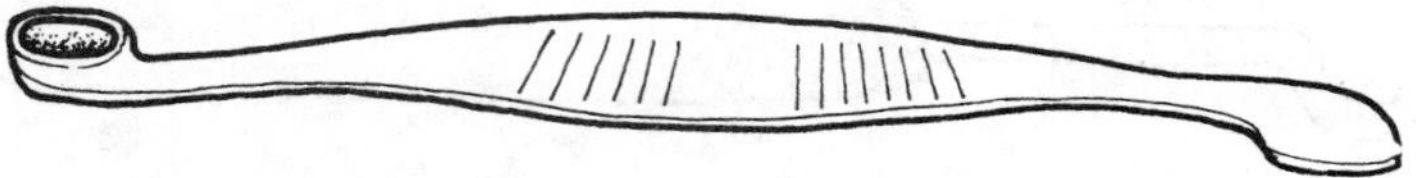

Figure 4.22 Volkmann curette or scoop

General instrument set

Once you have tried out all the different designs of available instruments, individual ones are chosen from each category. The chosen instruments are assembled into a 'general or standard set', which is a collection of instruments common to all operations likely to be performed. This set forms the basic nucleus; to it may be added further instruments needed for specific operations. It must be, when finished, a compact, inclusive unit.

It is important to decide at an early stage the composition of the general set, which should then be kept in a storage cupboard, always clean and available for an operation. Storage of the set as a single unit, with a card index documenting its contents, makes it easier to know exactly which instruments need to be sterilised before an operation, and to check at the end of an operation after cleaning that all instruments are present.

Every surgeon's general set is bound to vary but it is useful to have, for instance: artery forceps in a group of five; both sizes of knife handle; retractors of one's choice; and a pair each of medium and small sized scissors. A needle holder and a pair of forceps are also needed.

Cleaning

Following surgery, instruments are contaminated by blood, tissue, pus, etc., all of which put the person cleaning them at risk from cross infection.

This can be a cross infection from anything from a bacterial contamination to a virus infection, such as AIDs, and this risk must be explained to the person responsible for cleaning the instruments.

It is for this reason that the cleaning must be done while wearing heavy duty gloves rather than thin, surgical gloves. A mass of instruments tangled up in a bowl might easily tear a thin glove and traumatise the skin. With a thicker glove this is less likely.

Initially, having removed and discarded all the disposable 'sharps' such as knife blades, needles, etc., from amongst these dirty instruments, all the instruments are then rinsed in running water to remove the excessive contamination and then put in a bowl or sink containing Phoraid approximately 1 in 40.

Phoraid disinfectant is a rapidly acting disinfectant which is claimed to kill HIV, the AIDs virus, outside the body, as well as many other bacteria and viruses.

Each instrument is then individually washed and scrubbed well with a nail brush or tooth brush, particular care being taken to clean all the serrated surfaces and joints. They are then washed in clean water.

Following this they should be immersed in a solution of LUBE (Downs). This is a solution which protects the instruments against rust and also lubricates the joints.

From there the whole setting of instruments should be once again put through the autoclave and after a full cycle therein the instruments removed. The instruments, at this stage, because of the heat, virtually dry themselves.

If there is any residual moisture on them they can finally be dried off with a linen cloth and then put away for storage.

Care

Surgical instruments are precious tools and should be treated as such.

Artery forceps or haemostats are designed so that their jaws are just closed at a point when the ratchet is opposed at the other end, but the ratchet itself is not closed on its first notch.

This means, ideally, that they should be stored in this position so that the spring is not eased by perpetually being opposed against the ratchet. However, if the handle is just gently opposed, the ends do tend to fly open and this makes storage difficult. A compromise is usually reached where they are stored hung up with the finger-hole end closed on the first ratchet.

Dissecting forceps should be left open and not closed and held closed against the spring with an elastic band, as is occasionally the practice.

Tissue forceps can be closed on the first ratchet as the jaws are so designed that even at that point they are not opposed under tension.

Storage of instruments This will be discussed in more detail in the chapter on Theatre Area Design, but instruments should be stored in a dry space and always in 'sets'. This means that when put away each instrument has its own place and, at a glance, it can be confirmed that all the instruments that started the operation in the set are once more returned to it and that there are no gaps with the offending tool languishing in a dirty bin with soiled dressings ready to be thrown out at the end of the day.

If the system of 'sets' is used, then the preparation can be carried out by lay staff who sterilise a required set and do not have to know the individual instruments that should be included in any particular setting for any particular operation.

Instruments mellow and handle well with accurate use and real attention to their care. They deteriorate rapidly with bad care and improper use. Sometimes the moving parts should be lubricated with a 'silicone oil', especially after an enforced period of inactivity during vacation, etc.

CHAPTER 5

Disinfection and Sterilisation

Disinfection and bacterial sterilisation will now be discussed under three headings.

1. The Surgeon.
2. The Patient.
3. Instruments.

The surgeon — dress

In a full operating theatre all personnel of the surgical team are dressed in operating suits, antistatic footwear and wear a hat and mask. Following scrub-up when the hands and arms are cleaned they put on a sterile long-sleeved gown and sterile gloves.

In a minor operations theatre with no autoclaving facilities large enough to take gowns and linen for sterilisation, it is difficult to arrange for a sterile long-sleeved linen gown to be available for each case even though there are now very acceptable and comfortable prepacked and sterilised paper gowns.

However, the surgery to be performed is generally going to be:
(a) superficial, or
(b) should not take too long to complete.
This, put into the cost-effective equation, means that rather than wear an unsterile gown with long sleeves it is better to wear no gown at all, leaving the arms bare so that the surgeon has washed and scrubbed forearms and hands, which are technically clean, and is wearing sterile gloves.

As the surgeon is not covered by a gown and the patient is conscious under a local anaesthetic, the surgeon's dress is of paramount importance if the patient's confidence is to be maintained.

Normal trousers, shirt and rolled up sleeves and perhaps a neck tie tucked into the shirt to stop it hanging loose does the overall image of the surgeon no good. It also puts the surgeon's own clothes at risk and these can be protected only by wearing an apron. Once again this adds to the rather slipshod, macabre appearance implying that the surgeon anticipates the whole performance to be rather a bloody and hair-raising procedure.

Rather than wearing this type of outfit it is well worthwhile changing into a neat uniform. This either can be a set of one-coloured pyjamas with the sleeves of the jacket removed or a pair of dark linen trousers with short-sleeved shirt. It is much better to have the outfit coloured if possible.

If it is white it not only appears dirty at the slightest excuse but also any blood that is spilt does look like blood to the patient who sees it. With a dark outfit, it appears just as a wet patch. An apron with its inherent implications of anticipated incompetence should not be worn.

As antistatic shoes with local anaesthetic are not necessary, light, comfortable gym shoes appear better than the normal outdoor shoes which have been worn in the street. It does not take long to change and the bonus that it offers by converting the casual amateur uncertain appearance to that of the authoritative quietly professional, is well worth the small amount of trouble involved.

Cap and mask

As well as sterilising the skin of the hands and arms, the surgeon must also try to avoid contamination of the operative field with organisms transmitted there by himself. This can arise from organisms from his own nose or mouth but even more so from bits of contaminated dust or desquamated epithelial cells being shed from the surgeon's hair or scalp whilst operating.

Recent experimental work has shown the increased importance of adequate hair covering. Therefore, with all operative procedures the hair should be enclosed in a cap and a mask should also be worn.

In the past both the cap and the mask were made of linen which, after the operation, had to be washed and then re-sterilised.

The present-day disposable systems on the market offer convenience and availability and the modern design of paper from which the cap and mask is made is now so soft and supple that it is just as comfortable to wear as the old-time linen.

The paper from which the various designs of hats are made has some porosity, usually in the vault, which allows any perspiration to evaporate. There are various makes and styles and designs of hats which will vary in comfort depending upon the surgeon's personal preference and upon the type of hair style of the particular surgeon involved. It is suggested that the various styles be tried, noting the special features of enclosing as much of the hair as possible combined with a comfortable fit and a comfortable tying mechanism.

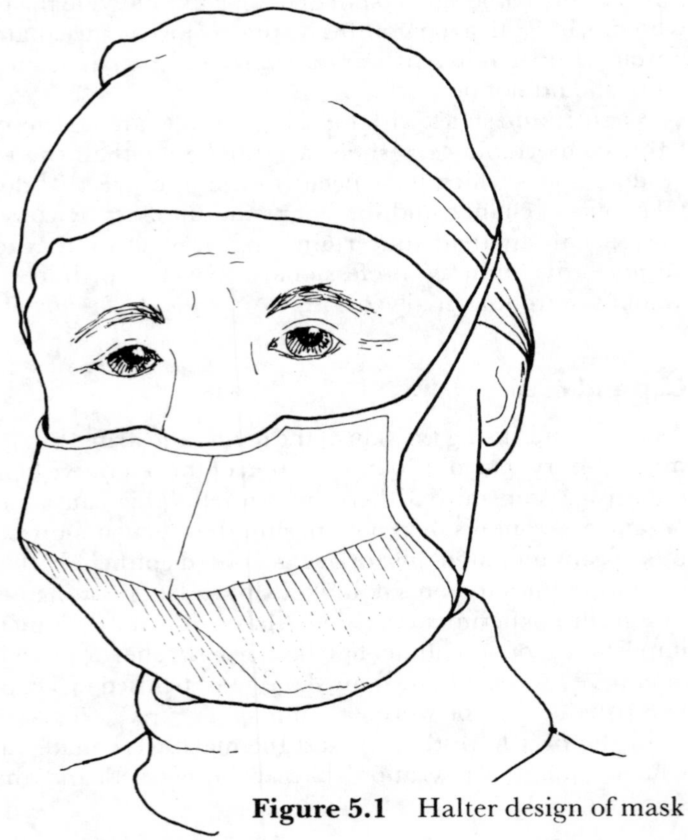

Figure 5.1 Halter design of mask

It is a good principle to have the cap lying down the forehead to about 3 cm above the eyebrows. Thus, if the temperature or tension rises during the surgery and the forehead starts to perspire, the moisture is mopped up by the rim of the hat and is neither obvious to the patient nor runs down the face to cause contamination problems by dropping in the sterile area.

As far as the design of the mask is concerned, this should certainly be of the halter design as in the diagram (Figure 5.1) rather than the old type of straight, flat mask which allows for considerable spill at the sides.

The disposable masks now normally have a flat thin band in the upper border which can be pressed around the nose and, having been so formed, retain their shape, creating quite a close fit. This is an important design feature especially for any surgeon who wears glasses as it tends to stop expired air being forced up under the mask and steaming up the glasses, but rather directs it out of the side of the mask as intended.

Needless to say, both the nose and mouth must be enclosed by the mask. In the past the practice of enclosing only the mouth where exhalation was supposed to occur and leaving the nose for theoretical sole inspiration is a practice that is not now accepted.

Having put on the hat and ensured that as much hair as possible is covered and enclosed by it, and also having adjusted the mask and carried out all the pre-scrub checks of trolley, materials and patients, etc., the surgeon is now ready to begin scrubbing-up.

The surgeon — scrubbing-up

The aim and object of scrubbing-up is to clean and, if possible, sterilise the skin of the hands and forearms up to the elbow.

Points about the actual scrubbing-up technique that perhaps should be emphasised are:

(a) The nails should always be trimmed on the short side of normal length.

(b) If there is any overt dirt under the nails this should be cleaned first of all with a normal nail file.

(c) Scrubbing-up should take place under running water and not in a bowl of static water.

(d) From the above this means that the surgeon scrubs up under a mixing tap where the hot and cold water combine and come out at one orifice. The volume and temperature of water is adjusted by long-handled taps which can be worked with the elbows and can be turned off when the scrub-up of hands and forearms is completed.

(e) When standing, either during or after scrubbing-up with the hands and arms wet, the hands must be held higher than the elbows so that any excess water runs down from the hands and off at the elbows rather than running from the elbows to the hands, i.e. from a potentially unsterile to a more sterile area.

(f) The substance used to scrub-up should be available in a dispenser which can be worked by a foot pump or elbow bar.

If soap of some sort is used, this should be kept in the hands from the start to the finish of the scrub up and not put down into a technically dirty soap holder, having to be lifted from that repeatedly during scrubbing-up.

(g) Whatever scrub-up material is used it must be used for the requisite length of time — as recommended by the manufacturers — for it be effective.

(h) The area cleaned must be from the elbow to the finger tips of both arms.

Antiseptic cleansing materials

For any antiseptic cleansing solution to be effective, it must be:

(a) Safe for routine use — to surgeon and patient.

(b) Have a low instance of sensitivity reaction against the surgeon's skin.

(c) Have a wide spectrum of antibacteriological activity.

(d) Have a rapid bacteriological activity against natural skin flora.

(e) If possible have some form of protection against accidental contamination later by leaving some protective antiseptic layer on the skin.

Of the different cleansing materials on the market it is considered that the choice lies between a chlorhexidine gluconate-containing solution, an iodine detergent formulation and, thirdly, a hexochlorophane emulsion or soap.

Chlorhexidine gluconate solution b.p. is found commercially in Hibiscrub which contains 4 per cent W/V chlorhexidine gluconate and Savlon which contains 1.5 per cent W/V of chlor-hexidine gluconate and also cetavlon cetremide b.p. 15 per cent W/V.

Hibiscrub After a one-minute wash with Hibiscrub with chlorhexidine gluconate at this strength, there is over 80 per cent kill against natural occurring skin flora, and cultures taken later show that this bacteriocidal activity is well maintained.

Savlon It does not have the high concentration of chlorhexidine gluconate but it has the advantage of having a powerful detergent combined with it. This means that this scrub-up is more useful if a surgeon's hands are greasy or have been contaminated with soil or dirt quite heavily before the operation and, as will be discussed later, it is a very useful combination for use in skin preparation for patients who come in following trauma.

Methods of use

Hibiscrub

Use undiluted. Wet the hands under constant running water, add about 5 ml of Hibiscrub from the dispenser and wash the hands and arms up to the elbows for one minute.

During this time, if required, a nail brush can be used for the finger nails. Rinse the ensuing lather off and repeat the wash for two minutes rinsing once again. During the second wash a nail brush should not be used unless it has been pre-sterilised.

Savlon

For scrubbing-up this must be used in a one-in-five dilution. Having had this solution made up, it is used in the same way with the same routine as the Hibiscrub.

Iodine detergent formulation

Free iodine has been known for many years to be a very powerful bacteriocidal agent but it is also known to have a high instance of irritating properties and sensitivity reactions.

However, if iodine is bonded to polyvinyl-pylrollidione there is, in effect, no elemental iodine present, but despite this the resulting solution maintains the bacteriocidal activity of the iodine whilst the sensitivity and irritating side effects of that drug are diminished.

Also, although the solution is the colour of iodine, this in fact is not an irremovable stain and can be removed by washing from any materials with which it comes in contact.

The percentage kill of natural skin flora after a one-minute wash is virtually equivalent to that of Hibiscrub but the long-term protection it offers is probably not significantly different.

Iodine detergent is marketed under the name of 'Disadine' and is used from a dispenser. The method of pre-operative use is as follows:

Wet the forearms and hands with water and apply about 3.5 ml of Disadine Surgical Scrub to the palm of the hands, spread over both hands and forearms. Rub the scrub over both hands using a brush if necessary for two minutes, paying particular attention to the finger nails. Add further water to develop a lather and rinse thoroughly under running water after a total of three minutes.

Post-scrub drying

Following the scrub-up, the hands and arms are dried with a sterile towel by first drying the hands and then moving to the arms and then discarding the towel. One must not start drying at the elbows and moving down to the hands as this increases the chance of contamination being carried down.

Hibiscrub, Disadine and Savlon are all products of I.C.I. and are marketed under those trade names.

The surgeon — gloving up

In theory, if a surgeon is wearing sterile gloves which have been put on with a non-touch technique, there should be no necessity for him to have to scrub-up and get the skin of his hands and his forearms as bacteria and spore-free as possible. However, it is so necessary for him to carry out this as on many occasions the gloves are breached either overtly or occultly, thereby bringing the operative field into direct contact with the skin.

Gloves

Glove size Glove size is determined before surgery by trial and error for each individual. It is important to get the length of the fingers from the web to the tip accurate. If the glove fingers are too long and the size too big there is a loose excess at the tip which makes accurate operating and touch impossible.

If the fingers are too short, there is a web at the proximal end in the glove which, on bending the fingers, makes it very restricting.

Having the fingers the right length, one then hopes that the glove itself is not too tight or too loose over the rest of the hand, but if there is any compromise to be made it should be in the fit of the hand rather than in the fit of the fingers.

Glove packaging Gloves made from latex by Puritee or Regent can be obtained pre-packed and sterile. When the outer pack is opened by an assistant or by the surgeon before scrubbing, the inner sterile pack can be dropped out onto the sterile trolley without being touched (Figure 5.2). The inner sterile pack is

Figure 5.2 Sterile glove packaging – opening packet to drop sterile glove onto sterile trolley

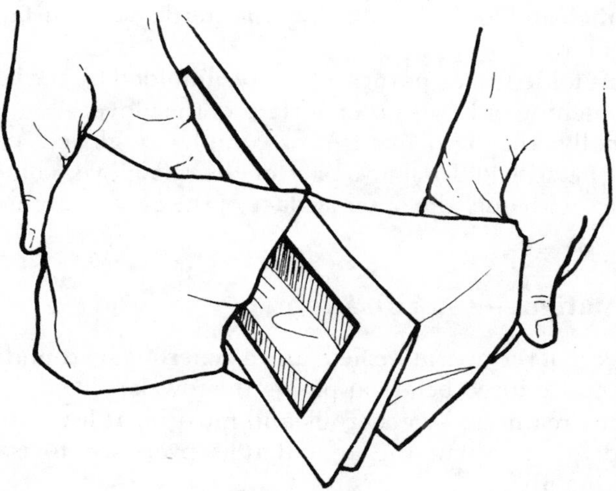

found to open like a wallet and inside is a small package containing the sterile lotion. In each side of the wallet lie the left and right hand glove. The gloves themselves are folded back at the wrist so that the opening where the hand is inserted is folded back onto itself.

Putting on the gloves The hands should be finally dried by using the sterile lotion pack which should be rubbed on both sides of the hands. Powder in open wounds has been shown to be a factor in fibrin and granulomatous formations so its use has been discontinued in favour of the lotion.

Procedure

The left glove is taken in the right hand by the fingers gripping the folded-over part of the glove and the left hand is then inserted and the glove pulled on. This means that the ungloved right hand is touching only that part of the left glove that is going to touch the skin of the left hand and wrist. The left-hand glove when on is left folded back on itself at the wrist.

Then the right glove is picked up by the already gloved left hand by sliding the fingers of that hand between the two layers of the folded back glove, thus coming into contact only with the clean surface of the glove. The right hand is pushed into the glove and the glove pushed on by the left hand so that the gloved clean hand contacts only the sterile outer surface of the right glove.

This folded-back part can then be unfolded by the left hand, still touching only the outer surface of the glove.

Finally, the right hand, now completely gloved, can push back the still folded back part of the left glove, coming into contact with only the outer surface of the glove. (Figures 5.2 to 5.7).

The patient — sterilisation

The skin of the operative field and a generous surrounding area must be sterilised before applying the towels.

The area must be generous and must be at least 10 cms all round greater than the area that is proposed to isolate by towelling up.

Figure 5.3 Sterile packet open. Inside of glove gripped with right hand as left is inserted, ie sterile surface not being touched

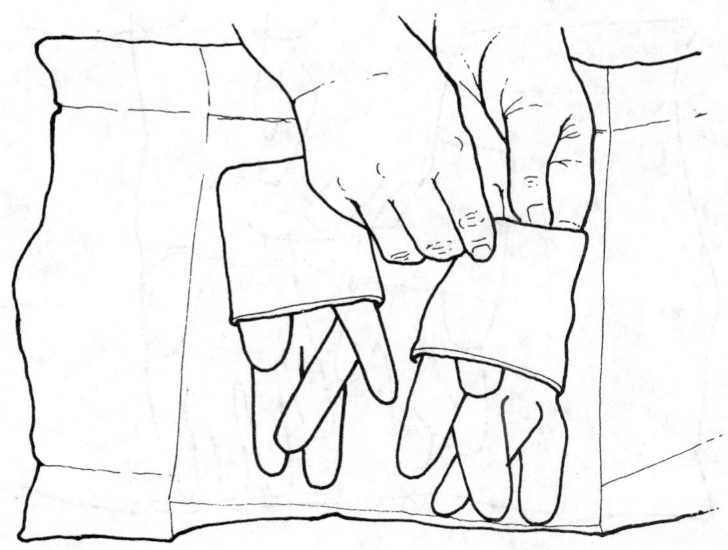

This means that there is a central area where the actual incision is to be made, a surrounding area which is enclosed by the towel but which is needed to be sterile for the identification of landmarks, ease of access etc., and then a further area which is sterile under the towels and overlapped by them for extra precautions to ensure that the central field is not going to be contaminated.

Cleaning the skin is a multiple exercise.

1. *Shaving.* Hairs should not only be shaved off, but the shaving must also be done well pre-operatively so that the loose hairs are removed.

   If the shaving can be done only pre-operatively then the loose hairs can be removed by dabbing the skin with the sticky side of elastoplast bandage to which the hairs will stick.

Figure 5.4 Left glove nearly fully on. When on, the overlapping upper flap is left folded

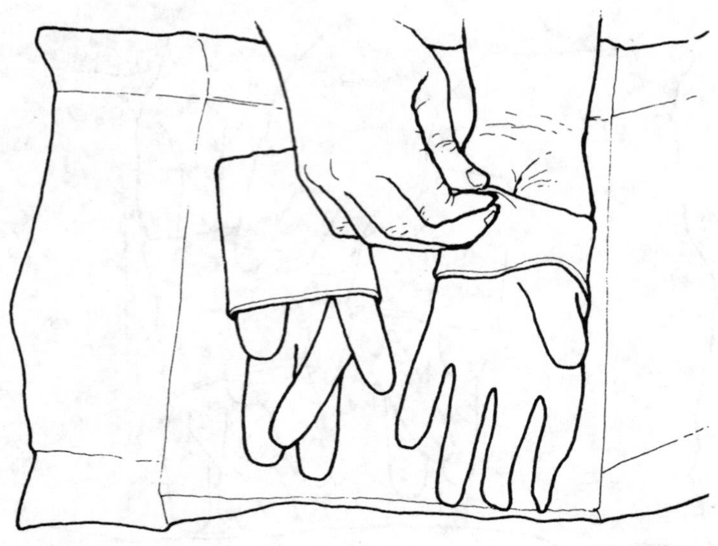

Figure 5.5 The right glove being pulled on by the clean left glove under the flap in contact with clean part of the glove

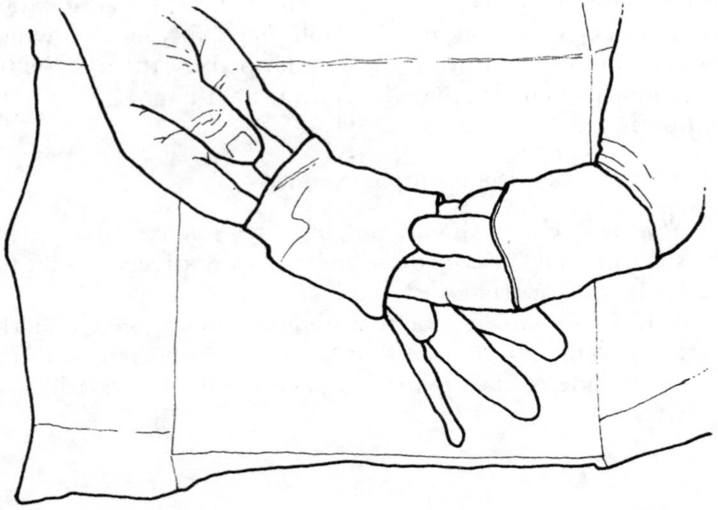

Figure 5.6 Right glove nearly on and flap turned down, still with left glove in contact with clean surface

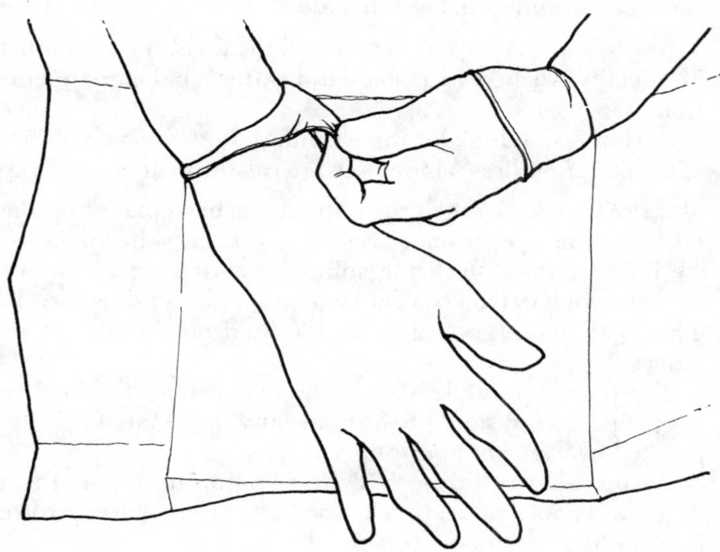

Figure 5.7 Right glove complete. Left glove now turned up with right hand in contact only with the clean external surface

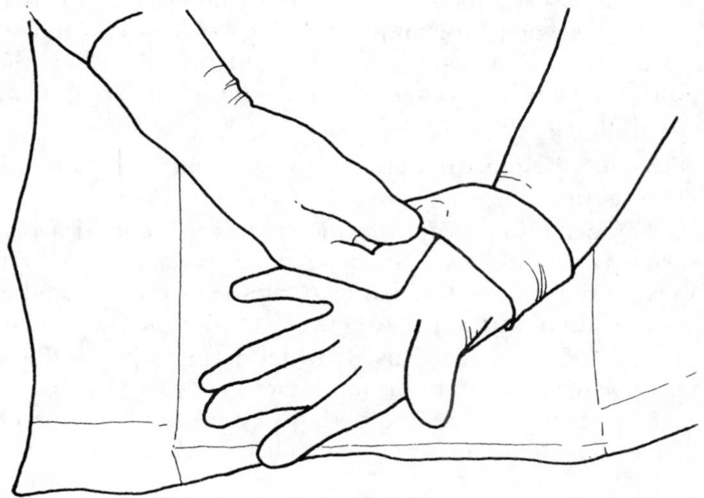

It is preferable not to shave rather than have loose hairs which cannot be removed and which might contaminate the incision and form foreign bodies.

2. *Socially clean.* After having shaved the area, the area must be socially washed with soap and water etc. before operation.

   Both the shaving and the washing are the responsibility of the patient unless it is obviously a case of an acute trauma.

3. *Skin sterilisation.* When the patient has been placed on the table and the operation is about to start, the skin should be sterilised with a sterilising solution carried on a swab or cotton wool ball which is held with a sponge holding forcep. This is to avoid getting excessive fluid on the operator's gloves.

   The paint up should start in the centre of the field where the proposed incision is to be made and then systematically painted, working out peripherally.

   Care should be taken that excess paint up does not run down and pool against the skin because prolonged exposure in this way may cause damage.

   Some paint ups are pigmented and some are clear.

   The advantage of the pigmented paint up, such as Betadine, is that the area that has been painted can be seen accurately. This avoids missing out any small sites.

   As will be explained later, the disadvantage of pigmented paint up is when a tourniquet is being used because it does fog up the visual assessment post-operatively when the tourniquet has been removed and the return of the capillary circulation has to be confirmed.

4. *Material.* Paint up materials may vary and are a matter of choice, but:

(a) As has been noted, if a tourniquet has to be used a pigmented paint up should not be used unless you are prepared to wipe that pigmented paint up off the skin at the end of the operation, with spirit, to get back the normal skin colour.

(b) If pure iodine is to be used, which is perhaps the most effective of all paint ups as far as sterilising the skin is concerned, then it is wise and perhaps essential to do a patch test for sensitivity on the patient. This should be done when the patient is first seen at the initial consultation, as a sensitivity reaction in this state is not infrequent and can result in both distress for the patient and worries for the surgeon.

Recommended paint ups:

(i) Standard Betadine — Similar but stronger than the Betadine Scrub already described. This is pigmented but can be cleaned from the skin with spirit.

(ii) Hibitaine in spirit — 0.5% Chlorhexadine which is non-pigmented or perhaps has a faint pink tinge which is acceptable if a tourniquet is being used.

Instruments — sterilisation

Micro-organisms which can cause pathology include bacteria and fungi and these are all killed by heat.

The heat to which they are exposed must be great enough and be kept at an acceptable level for an adequate length of time to bring about as near a one hundred per cent kill as possible.

This time factor is also related to the extent of the bulk of the contamination.

The most difficult of all the organisms to kill are the spores of clostridium and bacillus. If these can be destroyed it follows that all the other pathological micro-organisms will also be killed.

For years it has been assumed that boiling water was an adequate temperature. The time of emersion was related to the estimated time it took for the instruments to be brought up to the temperature of the boiling water, then maintained at that temperature for about five minutes.

Despite adequate times being allowed, the kill rate was not as effective as it could be, particularly in relation to the spores. The advent of the autoclave has now, therefore, replaced the boiling water steriliser.

The autoclave cycle of changes is related to the initial time that is taken to raise the temperature of the cold instruments to the pressure which can be achieved. The temperature and pressure are then held at that level for an adequate time. The pressure is then reduced and consequently the temperature so that cooling can take place, the autoclave opened and the instrument trays handled.

There is a variety of small autoclave units on the market, all of a very high quality and sophistication. They should be reviewed, remembering that the points to be considered are:

1. You need an adequate size of content space.
2. An adequate ease of usage.
   Ensure that you do not need an Honours Degree in electronics to work the machine.
3. Back up.
   It is most important to ensure that the back up provided by the company for servicing or emergency repair work is the best available.
4. Well-designed alarm and fail-safe features on the machine so that problems are brought to visible and audible notice if they arise.

Although there are many on the market that may be considered, perhaps you should always include the 'Little Sister 3' an admirable, well designed autoclave which runs off a 13 amp plug and complies with Health Technical Memorandum No. 10.

CHAPTER 6

Anaesthesia

J. B. Thomas, MB BCh DA FFARCS
Consultant Anaesthetist, Kent and Sussex Hospital
Tunbridge Wells, Kent

The purpose of this chapter is to describe simple, well-tried, local anaesthetic techniques with or without sedation to cover the surgical procedures, and to suggest a range of agents and equipment to carry them out. Monitoring, toxicity and its treatment will also be discussed.

Local anaesthetic agents

For our purposes, the range could be limited to three; Lignocaine (Xylocaine), Bupivacaine (Marcain) and Prilocaine (Citanest). Chemically they can be classified as amides and are degraded in the liver. Clearance rate is fastest with Prilocaine, then Lignocaine and slowest with Bupivacaine. Anaphylactoid-type reactions are extremely rare in these amide-linked drugs. Bupivacaine and Prilocaine are vasodilators, Lignocaine is neutral to the vessels.

The way in which local anaesthetic agents block nerve impulses is complex and not entirely worked out. They probably prevent depolarisation leading to non-conduction. Small non-myelinated fibres are the first to be affected, the sequence of block being autonomic, sensory and finally motor.

The injectable solutions are in the ionised state, but the agent is effective only in the non-ionised state. Thus the efficacy is dependent on the buffering effect of the tissues. This accounts for the difficulty experienced in using these agents in inflamed tissues and on mucous membranes where the buffering effects are low.

Lignocaine Hydrochloride BP (Xylocaine)

Suggested solutions 0.5 per cent, 1 per cent, 2 per cent.

Lignocaine 0.5 per cent and 1 per cent with Adrenaline 1:200,000

Preparations of 4 per cent strength are available for ophthalmic and mucous membrane anaesthesia.

Lignocaine is very stable and can be heated or autoclaved without decomposition. The 0.5 per cent and 1 per cent solutions, with or without adrenaline, may be used for infiltration; the 1 per cent or 2 per cent with or without adrenaline, for nerve block; and the 1 per cent or 2 per cent plain solution for finger blocks.

Lignocaine has also been used to suppress ventricular ectopic rhythm and has a mild central-sedative effect. Maximum safe dosage 7 mg/Kg with adrenaline, 3 mg/Kg without adrenaline.

Bupivacaine (Marcain, Marcaine)

Available in 0.25 per cent and 0.5 per cent solution, the 0.25 per cent solution being roughly equivalent to 1 per cent Lignocaine in action but of much greater duration, which is its principal advantage. Plain solutions can be repeatedly autoclaved, but solutions with adrenaline should not be heat sterilised more than twice.

Prilocaine (Citanest) — usual concentration 0.5 per cent

This agent is clinically and chemically very similar to Lignocaine, but is metabolised more quickly and widely in the body and, therefore, can be regarded as less toxic. It is most useful when a large dose of agent is required and is particularly useful in intravenous regional anaesthesia.

EMLA cream (Astra Pharmaceuticals)

This is a relatively recent innovation for topical anaesthesia of the skin. EMLA stands for 'eutectic mixture of local anaesthetics' and contains a 5% mixture of lignocaine and prilocaine in an oil-in-water emulsion.

When applied to intact skin in the directed amount and covered by an occlusive plastic dressing for 60–90 minutes, it produces local anaesthesia of the skin down to vein level. It is therefore very useful for painless intravenular injection, painless deeper injection of other local anaesthetic agents, and anaesthetising very superficial skin lesions prior to excision.

Adrenaline

This is the naturally occurring Alpha and Beta stimulating hormone with dramatic and widespread effects on the body when a threshold blood level is reached. It is usually used in a concentration of 1:200,000 in association with local anaesthetic agents producing local vasoconstriction and a relatively bloodless field. The restriction of the agent to the injected site results in a prolonged anaesthetic action with a lower peak concentration of the agent in the blood stream and, therefore, less liability to produce toxic symptoms.

However, it is not without problems on its own account — should the agent with adrenaline be inadvertently injected intravascularly, adverse and rapid effects may be produced, for example, tachycardia, ectopic rhythm, high B.P. and failing circulation, countered by the swift, intravenous injection of a Beta-blocker drug.

Some patients seem to be particularly sensitive to adrenaline and exhibit these effects with relatively low blood levels. It is best avoided in thyrotoxic or hypertensive patients and those individuals taking MAO's or tricyclic antidepressants.

It should not be used for ring blocks or the external ear when total cut off of the circulation is possible.

Toxicity of local anaesthetic agents

Toxicity is related to factors influencing serum level of drug, i.e. amount of solution injected, concentration, vascularity of injection site, use of adrenaline, rate of absorption and destruction, and size of patient, and to factors in the patient leading to increased susceptibility, e.g. age, fitness, cardiovascular disease, hypoxia.

Toxic reactions are primarily of two types and are typified by stimulation and depression of the cerebral cortex and medulla respectively.

1. Stimulation leading to nervousness, dizziness, blurred vision, nausea, tremors, convulsions and respiratory arrest.
2. Depression leading primarily to respiratory arrest, cardiovascular collapse and cardiac arrest. Symptoms can occur rapidly and with little warning.

Sedation

There is little doubt that a surgical procedure, however small, is made more tolerable and safe in the majority of patients by pre- or intra-operative sedation. It has to be said, however, that the use of sedatives means that more time has to be allowed for recovery, that the patient has to be accompanied home and must not drive during that day. There are a small number of patients who genuinely fear losing any lucidity of thought (or possibly its voluble expression). Despite temptation, it is unwise to persuade them to take a pill against their better judgement.

Suggested drugs

Pre-operative oral sedation is probably the best and only form necessary for children. It can conceivably be given at home before attending the surgery.

Trimeprazine tartrate given as Syrup Vallergan Forte (6 mg/ml) in a dose of up to 3 mg/Kg one to one-and-a-half hours pre-op. This phenathiazine derivative produces mild sedation, but presupposes the co-operation and parental preparation of the child. It is rarely necessary to exceed 15 mls of Syrup. Its relatively long action means that the patient will be sleepy for a few hours, probably not a disadvantage.

In adults it is hoped that pre-operative sedation can be avoided, but if thought necessary, use of a short acting benzodiazepine, Temazepam 10-20 mgm. Given one hour beforehand in the surgery, it should produce a calm patient.

Intra-operative intravenous sedation using Diazepam in the pain-free Diazemuls form, via a butterfly needle or cannula inserted on the non-operated side, can cover most situations, 10-20 mgs in an adult given in 5 mgm increments until the desired effect is produced. Although one of the longer acting benzodiazepines, when given intravenously, the duration of its action is not embarrassing provided that the amount injected is sufficient for use only as a sedative, and not a sleep-producing agent.

The patient

Certain groups of patients pose problems.

Children

For most surgery, general anaesthesia in hospital is to be preferred, but there is no doubt that local anaesthesia in properly controlled circumstances can be very successful, and a well-run dental practice bears testimony to this. Success relies on a good rapport beween practitioner, child and parent, a careful calm and confident approach, and an unhurried but expeditious technique. It is always a good ploy to tell the child how good he or she is, even if all the evidence is to the contrary.

If one does embark on local anaesthesia in children, it is essential to know the safe total dose of agents used for different ages and weights. Sedation, although unpredictable, is especially useful. Lastly, it is a wise practitioner who knows when to call a halt to proceedings in the case of an upset child. It is better to do this during attempted local anaesthesia rather than after surgery has started.

Patients with intercurrent disease

Whilst it may be tempting to carry out minor surgery on disabled patients who have difficulties in travelling to hospital, it is unlikely to be the safest way of dealing with the problem. Certainly those patients with conditions which lower the toxic threshold of local anaesthetic agents by cardiovascular problems, or respiratory disease associated with hypoxia, are best avoided. Similarly, those individuals with unusual medical conditions, e.g. rare genetic disorders where the ramification of treatment is unknown, are best dealt with in a hospital setting.

Nervous and frightened patients

A small amount of sedation may help, but it may not, and one has to bear in mind that complications are likely to be more common in these patients, e.g. arrythmias, nausea, vomiting.

Assessment and general pre-operative preparation

The patient's General Practitioner will be in an excellent position to know the relevant medical background, present medical condition and treatment, and past problems. These will be of importance in relation to local anaesthetic agents and sedation. Previous experience of operation and anaesthesia may well influence the choice of technique. Sensitivity and allergy to drugs, skin-cleansing agents and adhesive tape, etc., may be noted. The most important aspect of preparation is the rapport between the patient and doctor and the full explanation of all intended procedures.

Those patients who are going to have an elective surgical procedure under local anaesthetic in contradistinction to the emergency cases of trauma, have usually been for consultation and their condition diagnosed and surgery suggested.

The patient may be apprehensive and nervous at the thought of surgery, and it is vitally important that this apprehension and worry should be allayed.

At the initial consultation it is important to give the patient a brief but detailed explanation of the routine and sequence of events to expect when he returns for surgery.

It is recommended that a light meal only should be permitted three hours beforehand and, after that, drinks only as required, in order to try to ensure that the stomach is empty, thus diminishing the possibility of nausea and perhaps vomiting in a nervous patient.

Shaving should be carried out by the patient on the evening preceding the proposed date for surgery. The area to be shaved around the proposed operative site should be marked out on the patient's skin with an indelible skin pencil by the doctor at the first consultation. This ensures that the patient is in no doubt as to the area to be cleared. If this is in an inaccessible site, obviously he or she will have to arrange for a friend or one of the family to shave the area for them. If this is impossible and the surgery nurse is available, it is better for the patient to be shaved the previous evening by her at the surgery, rather than for the doctor to have to do the shaving immediately before the operation.

If it has to be done pre-operatively by the doctor, it should preferably not be done in the clean surgical area. Apart from the time element, the disadvantage of this is that inevitably loose hairs are still around which will add to the risk of sepsis. There is also the risk of these hairs falling into the wound and creating a foreign-body reaction. Also, if the shaving is done immediately pre-operatively, the after-shave wash has to be foregone.

The best method for removing loose hair following a shave is to get an approximate 20 cm length of 5 to 8 cm Elastoplast. By holding the ends in either hand and stretching the Elastoplast between them, it can be repeatedly pressed sticky side down over the shaved area and any loose hairs stick to the strapping and are removed.

If the patient has shaved himself the previous evening, the area, following the shave, should be washed very thoroughly to remove any loose hairs. If possible some form of antiseptic soap should be used.

Intra-operative care

Despite the simplicity of local anaesthetic procedures, the increasing standard of patient care requires a level of continuing clinical observation and monitoring which would now be regarded as mandatory. In addition, an ability both in terms of skill and equipment to deal with the complications of such anaesthesia up to and including circulatory arrest, should be available. Before dismissing these requirements as too arduous, it is worth reflecting that these facilities might reasonably be expected of any doctor in his surgery.

Practical approach to observation and monitoring

One other competent person, apart from the operator, should always be present and should not be involved in preparation work etc. when the operation is in progress, but be available to observe, monitor and, if appropriate, converse with the patient. General clinical observation will include demeanour, colour, pulse, B.P., and respiratory rate.

Monitoring

ECG. The simplicity and relatively low cost of the recent generation of these small screen monitors make them most worthwhile and useful. Three stick-on, upper chest electrodes allow continuous observation of electrical activity of the heart, seeing pulse rate changes and any arrythmias immediately, especially important in relation to toxic effects of local anaesthetic agents and adrenaline.

Administration of local anaesthetic

With the patient correctly positioned on the couch and the light adjusted, the instrument trolley is checked. The surgeon — having scrubbed and put on his gloves — then cleans the operative area, and puts the appropriate towels in place.

The cap of the multidose local anaesthetic bottle is then cleaned with the same solution as just used for the skin preparation. The swab used to clean it is then discarded.

A drawing-up needle on the syringe is then inserted through the cap of the bottle and, having checked that the bottle in fact contains the correct anaesthetic solution in the correct strength — plain or with adrenaline — the appropriate amount is drawn up into the syringe.

Despite the amount of local anaesthetic needed, a 20 ml syringe should always be used, even if only 5 ml is drawn up into it. This practice cuts down the risk of inadvertently picking up from the trolley a syringe containing some other clear fluid, such as sclerosant for the injection of varicose veins, and mistaking it for local anaesthetic. All the other fluids discussed under 'Surgical Techniques' will be drawn up in smaller syringes. Thus, any 20 cc syringe on the trolley should contain only local anaesthetic.

Drawing the local anaesthetic out of the bottle is sometimes made easier by injecting the same amount of air into the bottle as the contents one wants to withdraw.

When sufficient local anaesthetic is in the syringe, it is then detached from the drawing-up needle, which is then removed from the bottle cap by the assistant, and then discarded.

A new, fine-bore needle is then attached to the syringe and anaesthesia can be started.

Local anaesthetic for the surgery proposed can be classified into the following groups:

1. Local infiltration
2. Nerve block
(a) Intravenous block
(b) Hand blocks
(c) Digital blocks

The technique of administration of these local anaesthetics will now be discussed.

Local infiltration

The area of anaesthesia required must be large enough to surround the incision that is to be made. It must also extend laterally from the line of the intended incision to allow for the final sewing-up of the skin, so that the area of insertion of the skin stitches lateral to that incision is also anaesthetised.

(a) The layer of infiltration — subcutaneous.

(b) The skin is punctured by the needle. No intracutaneous bleb injection is needed as this is much more painful than the actual injection of the anaesthetic itself.

(c) Before injecting, the needle should be aspirated to check it has not inadvertently punctured a blood vessel.

(d) A half to 1 ml of whichever anaesthetic is being used is injected and then a pause is held before further injection to check that the patient is not reacting to or is sensitive to the anaesthetic agent.

(e) If there is no reaction, the local anaesthetic is injected ahead of the slowly advancing needle. By so doing, this cuts down the risk of puncturing a vessel as it tends to be swept out of the way by the fluid.

(f) The areas to be anaesthetised and the order of so doing is illustrated below.

When one-quarter segment is infiltrated, the needle is all but withdrawn and then rotated through 90° to infiltrate the second segment.

The two further segments can then be infiltrated by the needle being put through an already anaesthetised segment of skin at the apex of the two previous infiltrations. (Figure 6.1.)

(g) If infiltration is carried out with a local anaesthetic containing a vasoconstrictor, a very good estimate of the area that has been anaesthetised is quite often obtained by the degree of skin pallor due to skin vessel vasoconstriction that occurs soon after the infiltration is carried out.

Resume

In order for a local anaesthetic infiltration to be satisfactory, remember:

1. Infiltrate in the right place and tissue plane.
2. Infiltrate an adequate area.

3. Above all give the anaesthetic time to work before starting any surgery.

Figure 6.1 Infiltration anaesthesia

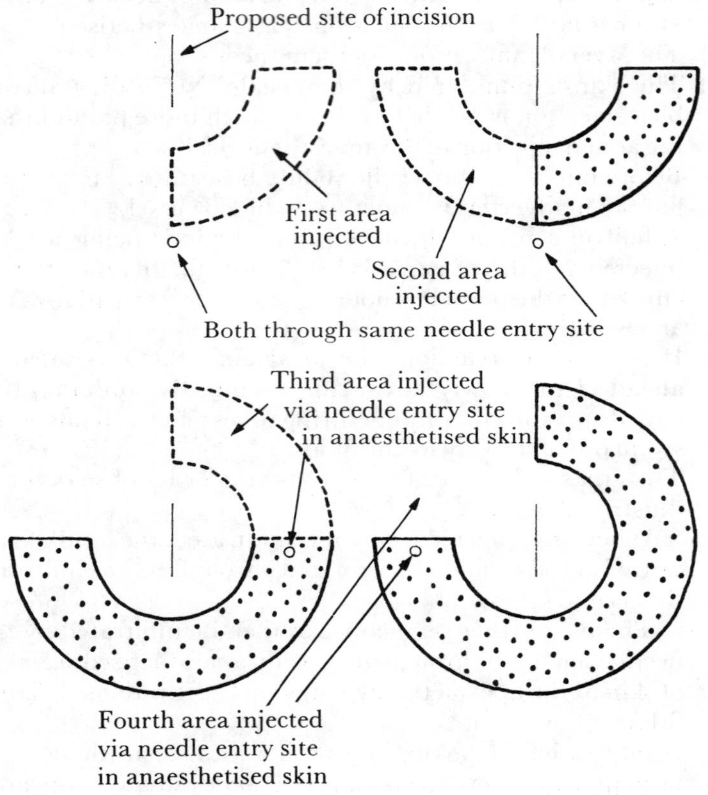

Nerve block

(a) **Intravenous block**

This method is best confined to the arm where it is possible to achieve excellent anaesthesia and bloodless field of hand, wrist and lower forearm. Anaesthesia of the upper forearm and elbow are less predictable.

It relies on the retrograde flow using a large volume of low concentration of anaesthetic agent into a tourniqued and exsanguinated limb, thus blocking the peripheral nervous system at the nerve endings. Despite using a low concentration, the total dose may approach toxic levels so it is vital to confine the agent to the limb for at least ten minutes when it is expected that the major part of it will have become fixed in the tissues.

Research has shown that there is, unfortunately, no absolutely safe minimum tourniquet time and it is, therefore, important to be on the alert for toxic effects after the tourniquet is released.

Prilocaine is now regarded as the agent of choice for this procedure because it is less liable to produce toxic effects following relatively high dosage.

Contra-indications for the technique would include Raynaud's disease, sickle cell anaemia and scleroderma.

Technique

An intravenous cannula is inserted into the non-operated arm for access to the circulation and an ECG monitor is set up. A butterfly needle, or small plastic cannula, is inserted into one of the dorsal veins of the hand of the side to be anaesthetised. The tourniquet is applied to the upper arm, uninflated. It should be of the purpose-made (orthopaedic) type with bicycle-type pump, and regularly checked. The limb is elevated until blanching is evident. Further exsanguination is produced by brachial compression or the use of an Esmarch bandage wound from fingers to lower border of tourniquet. The tourniquet is inflated to 200 mmHg and the time noted. The Esmarch, if used, is now removed.

In adults, 30 to 50 mls of 0.5 per cent Prilocaine is injected through the previously placed needle or cannula. Anaesthesia soon follows and the patient is ready for operation in approximately 10 to 15 minutes.

Time of operation is limited to discomfort of the tourniquet which may start after 15 minutes and slowly increase in intensity, so the technique is best used for operations of less than 20 minutes duration.

Dressings and outer crepe-type bandage are applied before release of the tourniquet.

(b) **Hand blocks**

Ulnar, radial and median nerve blocks

These techniques have the advantage for relatively confined areas of anaesthesia, but without the advantage of a bloodless field and muscular relaxation expected with an intravenous block.

Ulnar nerve block

The cutaneous sensory nerve element of the ulnar is distributed to the hand in the areas depicted in Figure 6.2. Thus it can be seen that the little finger is the only one that can be virtually guaranteed to be totally anaesthetised with this block. If the ring or middle finger are needed to be operated upon, this block must be augmented with a median or radial block as well.

Technique

Agent — 10 ml, 1 per cent Lignocaine should be drawn up in a 20 ml syringe, the drawing-up needle discarded and a fine needle put into its place.

Surgical anatomy

The ulnar nerve at the level of the wrist lies lateral to the tendon of the flexor carpi ulnaris which runs down the ulna border of the arm and is inserted into the pisiform bone.

The ulna nerve can quite often be palpated lying lateral to this tendon before its insertion into the pisiform.

After cleaning the skin, a small wheal is raised and the needle inserted at right-angles to the skin, lateral to the tendon over the nerve.

When the needle has gone through the deep fascia, before the injection, quite often there is a feeling of parasthesia due to contact with the nerve.

Once the needle is in the correct position about 5 ml of the 1 per cent Lignocaine is injected.

The dorsal sensory branch of the ulna nerve supplying the back of the hand quite often leaves the nerve more proximal than this block and, therefore, in order to ensure that the dorsal nerve is blocked as well, a sub-cutaneous injection should be carried out of a further 5 ccs of 1 per cent Lignocaine from the

Figure 6.2 Distribution of the cutaneous sensory nerve element of the ulnar

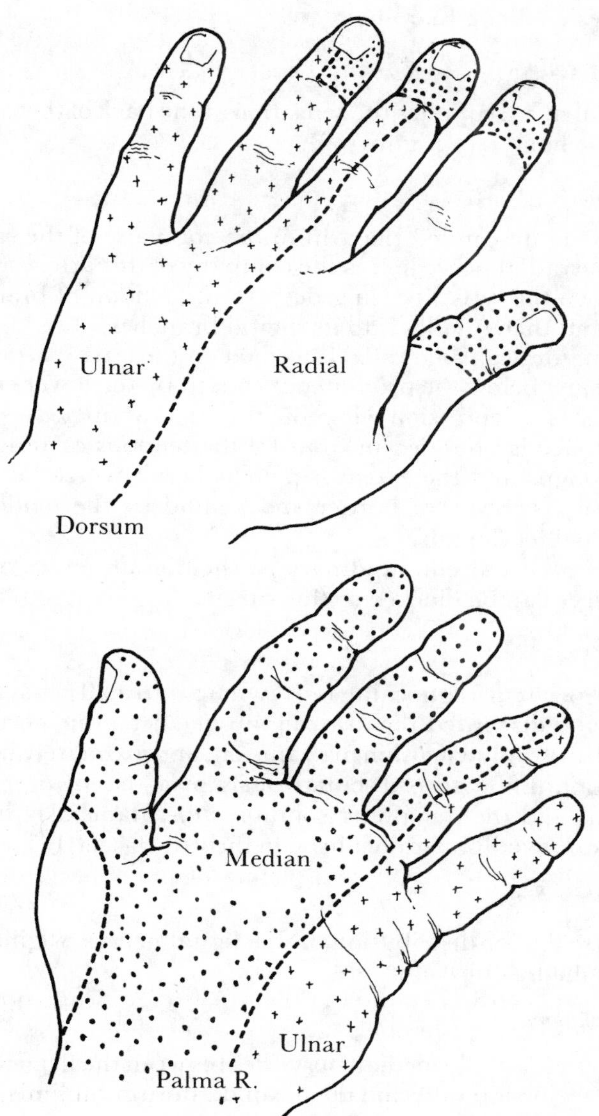

medial side of the tendon of the flexor carpi ulnaris at the level of the ulna syloid process to the middle of the back of the wrist. This is carried out, as previously described under 'Infiltration Anaesthesia', along that line.

Radial nerve block

The radial nerve supplies the sensation at the back of the lateral part of the hand (see Figure 6.2).

Surgical anatomy

After having descended the arm in the company of the radial artery, the radial nerve leaves the company of this artery about 7 cm above the wrist, passing deep to the tendon of brachio-radialis and then divides into its digital branches.

The anatomical 'snuff box' is formed on the lateral aspect of the wrist just below the prominence caused by the lower end of the radius as a depression when the thumb is abducted.

This space is bounded in front by the tendons of abductor pollicis longus and the extensor pollicis brevis which lie close together on its anterior border and behind by the tendon of extensor pollicis longus.

This is a very useful landmark as the digital nerves of the radial nerve can be blocked at this site.

Technique

5 ccs of 1 per cent Lignocaine is drawn up into a 20 ccs syringe and, having discarded the drawing-up needle, a fine needle is attached and, following skin preparation, approximately half of the solution infiltrates sub-cutaneously over the lower end of the radius and the remaining solution sub-cutaneously in the anatomical 'snuff box' previously described.

Median nerve block

See Figure 6.2 for distribution of the digital nerves originating from the median nerve.

Surgical anatomy

At the wrist joint, the median nerve lies between the flexor carpi radialis tendon laterally and the flexor digitorum sublimis, with the palmaris longus tendon medially.

The nerve lies deeply between these two tendons and cannot usually be palpated.

Technique

After having drawn up 5 ml of 1 per cent Lignocaine in a 20 ccs syringe and having discarded the drawing-up needle and replaced it with a fine infiltration needle, the skin is sterilised and cleaned around the wrist. The landmarks previously described are made prominent by flexing the wrist against tension, making the tendons stand out.

The palmaris longus tendon is a variable feature, sometimes not being very prominent.

The needle is inserted and if parasthesia in the nerve distribution is elicited the injection is carried out at that time and in that area but if this does not occur, injection is carried out moving the needle point slightly laterally and medially while so doing to ensure a wider spread.

Resume

In order to get the best possible results with local anaesthetic of any type it is essential that:

1. Pre-operative anxiety is relieved with adequate, well-timed sedation.
2. A good rapport is obtained with the patient to gain his confidence and co-operation.
3. There is no haste or fluster. Everything is done step by step with quiet confidence, dexterity and skill.
4. Each successive move is explained to the patient before it is carried out.
5. All the relevant neuroanatomy of whichever block is being used is known beforehand.
6. The possible complications of the local anaesthetic being used are known and the treatment for them is immediately available if they should arise.
7. If an assistant is present that person should be conversant with the procedure being undertaken. Excessive instructions and questions quickly destroy the patient's confidence which has taken time to build up.
8. If supplementary analgesia or sedation are needed they must be readily available.

9. All the requirements for the actual operation are checked and ready so that the surgery can start in a quietly controlled, competent way, without any fuss and at the optimum time from the anaesthetic point of view.

(c) **Digital blocks**

This technique is used to anaesthetise a digit of either finger or toe, the nerve supply to which is a palmar and dorsal digital nerve on each side of the digit, all of which have to be blocked to establish anaesthesia of the digit.

Contraindications

1. On no account must any local anaesthetic agent containing adrenaline or adrenaline-like vasoconstrictor substance be used.
2. It is a good principle to have at least one phalanx distance between the site of the block and any infection, if the block is being done for this pathology.

   Thus, with a pulp or sub-ungual infection or paronychia of the thumb, it is risky to be doing a digital block as there is an increased hazard of the block site becoming infected.
3. Raynaud's or severe vaso-spastic disease.
4. Scleroderma.

Surgical anatomy (See Figure 6.3.)

Figure 6.3 Diagrammatical cross-section of digital block

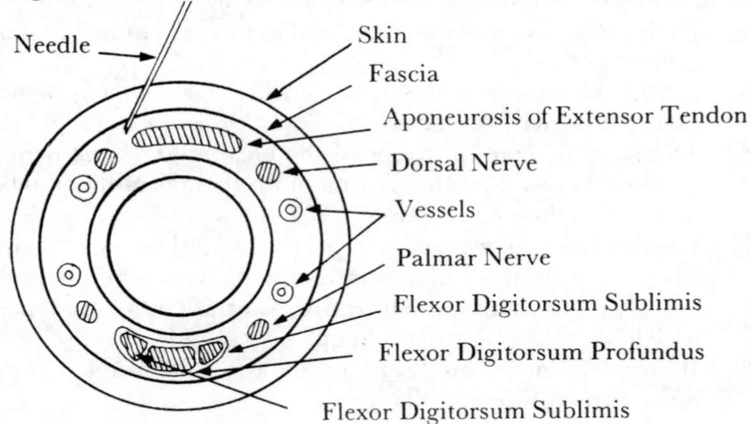

Technique

Agent — 1 per cent Lignocaine with no adrenaline. Approximately 5 ccs to be drawn up in a 20 ccs syringe and having rejected the drawing-up needle, a fine bore needle attached to the syringe.

Method

A wheal is raised over the dorsum of the base of the proximal phalanx of the digit to be anaesthetised after cleansing of the skin.

Through the centre of this intra-cutaneous wheal the needle of the syringe is inserted in a palmar direction, keeping close to the side of the phalanx at its base and injecting as the needle is advanced until the end of the needle has virtually reached the palmar skin.

During the advancement of the needle approximately 2 ccs is injected on that side.

The needle is then withdrawn until it is virtually out of the puncture hole in the wheal and is then advanced in a similar manner through the same entry site, injecting ahead of its advancement as before down the other side of the base of the phalanx to the same depth.

Following injection it is normal practice to put a small rubber tourniquet around the digit at the injection site and at least five minutes must elapse to enable the injection and block to work before any surgical procedure is started.

Problems of local anaesthesia

The philosophy of dealing with iatrogenic troubles related to local anaesthesia can be considered under the following headings:

1. Avoiding trouble
2. Early treatment of problems
3. Being prepared to deal with circulatory arrest

Avoiding trouble

(a) Keeping well within known toxic levels of drugs
Maximal recommended dosage:

	Plain	*With Adrenaline*
Lignocaine Hydrochloride	3 mg/Kg	7 mg/Kg
Bupivacaine	2 mg/Kg	—
Prilocaine	10 mg/Kg	—

(b) Using a technique likely to minimise intravascular injection — moving the needle and frequently aspirating.

(c) In intravenous regional anaesthesia using checked and faultless tourniquet equipment and a strict adherence to minimum tourniquet time before its release.

(d) In intravenous sedation using small initial dosage and increments to achieve the desired effect and waiting for a minute or so after each injection.

Early treatment of problems

This assumes good observation and monitoring and that a competent third party is present to help. Should any untoward signs appear during the injection of the local anaesthetic agent, then the administration should cease.

If there is any unexpected change in conscious level, observation or ECG during the procedure, the surgeon should stop and take stock of the position.

Access to the circulation with an intravenous cannula for both fluids and drugs (e.g. Venflon 16 or 18) is vital. Central nervous stimulation, particularly associated with muscular twitching, requires immediate use of sedation with Diazepam (Diazemuls) in 5-10 mg increments.

Any element of circulatory failure — hypotension and poor peripheral circulation — is treated with a rapid intravenous infusion of N. Saline 250-500 mls before re-assessment and repeating if necessary. 100 per cent oxygen should be given via a face mask. Bradychardia must be assumed to be due to hypoxia and treated with oxygen initially but atropine 0.6 mg intravenously repeated if necessary, will raise the pulse rate in most cases.

Tachycardia of over 120, especially if accompanied by ectopic rhythm, particularly of multifocal type and with good peripheral circulation, could be reasonably thought to be due to circulating adrenaline either injected or endogenous and treated with a Beta-blocker (e.g. Propanolol (Inderal) ½-1 mg I.V.), but particular care should be taken with asthmatic patients.

Respiratory depression, either in rate or depth, should be treated by assisting or taking over the ventilation with bag, mask and valve arrangement and oxygen.

Allergic phenomena using the suggested local anaesthetic agents are extremely rare, but would require antihistamines, steroids and I.V. fluids.

Being prepared to deal with circulatory arrest

Individual practitioners must decide how much provision they are prepared to invest in a resuscitation regime available to deal with iatrogenic and primary circulatory inadequacy and arrest.

Treatment of circulatory arrest requires a level of organisation, skill and equipment that ideally would be present in a health centre and group practice surgery. It is more than likely that the Practitioner enthusiastic enough to set up a minor surgery service would also rise to meet this particular requirement.

The skills

Chest compression (external cardiac massage), is probably familiar to all, but requires some training to optimise cardiac output and minimise organ damage.

Skills of airway control, lung inflation with mask, bag and valve arrangement, and possibly endotracheal intubation can probably best be acquired with an anaesthetist during the course of routine operating lists in a hospital. Intubation, whilst ideal, is by no means essential for lung inflation and is a skill that takes time to acquire.

The equipment

Oxygen cylinder, reducing valve and flowmeter
Mask, bag and valve arrangement
Airways
Suction apparatus, electrical or foot operated
I.V. cannulae
I.V. fluids

Drugs

All drugs likely to be required can be commercially obtained in a single sealed pack, changeable after each use and time expiry. (See page 14.)

D.C. defribillator

The most expensive item, but today eminently small, portable and simple to use, with incorporated ECG monitor.

The organisation

This should ensure:

1. The availability of sufficient people with skills, knowledge of equipment and its location, to set resuscitation in motion at any necessary time.
2. A programme for checking and changing drugs and equipment.
3. Written instructions and arrangements for documentation.

Technique

The chance of success will be greatest on early recognition and immediate instigation of effective treatment.

Diagnosis

1. ECG monitoring on all patients undergoing any surgical or anaesthetic procedure will quickly alert those involved to problems and enable them to make a definitive diagnosis of the type of arrest — asystole or ventricular fibrillation.
2. Loss of consciousness and cadaveric facial appearance.
3. Dilation of pupils.
4. Absence of pulse, radial, carotid and femoral.

Treatment

1. Call 'Help' and start cardiac arrest drill and ring bell.
2. Instigate and continue external cardiac massage with patient on flat and firm surface.
3. Instigate and continue inflation of lungs with oxygen, sucking out pharynx if necessary.
4. Set up intravenous infusion using cannula already *in situ*, 100 mmols sod. bicarbonate should be given first.
5. Set up ECG monitor if not attached, to diagnose type of arrest.

Cardiac massage and lung inflation will have to be continued until adequate circulation and respiration returns. If the heart is in asystole, adrenaline 0.5–1.0 mg is given I.V. or even directly into the heart. If the response is inadequate, the adrenaline is repeated in two minutes and calcium chloride 10 mls of 1 per cent solution may also be injected. This treatment may produce a heartbeat and output, but might well produce ventricular fibrillation (V.F.)

Primary V.F. may also be treated with adrenaline 0.05-0.2 mg to increase the rate and amplitude of fibrillatory waves as seen on ECG, which gives a much better chance of reverting to a satisfactory rhythm and output on defibrillation.

Defibrillation

D.C. shock across the heart, properly applied and with due precaution, it is hoped, will convert V.F. to a rhythm which will provide a measurable cardiac output. A single shot of 100 watt-seconds increasing to 400 watt-seconds are the usual settings.

Continuing treatment may well be necessary. Ionotropic stimulation with Isoprenaline may now suffice and will be expected to increase greatly pulse rate and output. Ionotropic stimulation, together with vasopressor effect, can be produced by use of Dopamine infusion 5 mg in 500 mls until the B.P. comes up to a normal level.

If a reasonable cardiac output is achieved as judged by pulse, B.P. and returning consciousness, transfer of patient to hospital for further treatment is now undertaken.

CHAPTER 7

General Principles of Surgical Techniques

This will be discussed under the general headings of:

1. Introduction and handling of tissue.
2. Haemostasis.
3. Principles of tissue healing and repair.

Introduction and handling of tissue

Any surgical procedure carried out on a patient constitutes a physical insult and is an attack on the integrity of the organism.

It is only a matter of degree whether the insult to the tissues is one caused by the most delicate and beautifully performed operation, or is one of open agricultural brutality.

The insult begins at the time the skin is breached with the needle and the tissues separated, as the local anaesthetic agent is injected, and it ends several days later when the stitches are removed.

The insult can be minimised by many factors. A competent, precise technique where one cut is used instead of three with a resulting lessening of trauma.

This surgical confidence comes with experience and is not only reflected in the actual mechanics of the procedure but also radiates itself out and is felt by the patient whose anxiety and apprehension is diminished and who then consequently is more relaxed, which in turn makes the surgery easier and, by so doing, makes it less traumatic.

The handling of tissue with understanding and thought, where tissue is not dragged and hauled around, but is caressed with the instrument, whether it be a retractor, a knife, or simply the fingers, which must be used delicately and with respect.

Tissue plains are carefully identified and opened by stroking and teasing with a sharp blade rather than tearing and pulling apart with a gauze swab used in the fond and erroneous belief that it stands less chance of causing damage if one is not quite certain about the position of surrounding tissues.

Using a gauze swab is a technique which may be used on a very few occasions in specific instances, but as a general technique it must be considered to be the haven of the surgically destitute as its whole basis is one of tearing and traumatising tissue.

Too-heavy handling and resulting trauma to the tissues is reflected during surgery by oedema or bruising, and if this is severe it is not just microscopic but can be seen, and when it reaches that stage is a pure endictment of bad technique.

Instruments have been designed, redesigned and modified many times over the years, to have developed to their present design. No doubt over years to come they will be further changed and honed to try to seek more and more improvement.

Each instrument is a precise tool developed for a specific purpose and that purpose is well delineated, and within those parameters the particular tool reigns supreme. Start using that tool outside its design intention and both the instrument and the tissue suffer. For instance, cutting skin with the shearing action of scissors rather than the precise atraumatic cut of a knife blade not only tends to spring the jaws of the scissors, but also traumatises the tissue in a marked and unacceptable way. Holding a corner of a swab with a delicate artery forceps to blot some oozing vessel springs the joint of the instrument and the next time it is used to clip a vessel that vessel will slip.

Using instruments to hold tissue, which are not designed for that purpose, and which have to exert their hold on the tissue by a crushing pressure, causes tissue damage and impaired healing.

Speed of surgery is important. To rush means there is a larger likelihood of running into problems which slow down procedure, whereas if one is slow and pernickety and indecisive, the tissue gets a bit oedematous, the exposure is longer, the anaesthetic wears off a little and suddenly the whole performance becomes rather fraught instead of being totally under control.

Being a fast and slick operator is a tag which may be sought by the young and inexperienced, but the unhurried, calm and controlled surgeon, who maybe takes a few minutes longer over the operation, begets a better result for the remaining years of the patient's life, and this is what should be sought.

It is sometimes permissible in life to fool friends or patients, but, as a surgeon, never fool oneself, as that is a recipe for disaster. Surgeons must try to develop insight and self-critical analysis as to the competence of their efforts and, by doing so, a correct balance for each individual, of speed against ability, will emerge.

It is my belief, for instance, that the removal of stitches post-operatively should be done by the surgeon who performed the operation and not delegated to a nurse or someone else. This is for many reasons ranging from the surgeon/patient relationship, which is then further consolidated, down to surgeons being able to see the early stages of the end result of their efforts.

It is only right that surgeons should get the lift that really successful operations and scars produce, allied to the pleasure and satisfaction of the patients with the result. It is also important that if the result is not quite so good as the surgeon would have wished there is the opportunity to learn from it for the next time. It is an addition to experience, but possible only if the surgeon has developed the honest, self-critical analysis that is needed.

A surgeon has the privilege of dealing with living tissue but with that privilege the surgeon must, all the time, be conscious of the responsibility that accompanies it.

With surgery, the surgeon must be firm yet gentle, as a mother with her child, caressing the tissue with understanding and precision, and if this is done it will respond with a healing beautiful to behold.

Haemostasis (or arrest of bleeding)

During surgery bleeding occurs from tissue by cutting or traumatising:

1. Fine capillaries.
2. Visible vessels, either small veins or arteries.

Fine capillary bleeding

When any tissue is cut there is capillary oozing. This is coming from vessels too fine to secure with instruments and this bleeding will stop due to vessel spasm. The application of pressure, maintained for an adequate time — with or without heat — encourages this to occur.

Pressure can be applied directly by the surgeon pressing the area with a moist swab or, alternatively, by packing the area tightly with a swab and leaving it in place for a few moments.

In either case the essential ingredient is time. Bleeding will not stop and remain stopped with only a few seconds pressure and a prayer.

It is a very good exercise for the surgeon to apply pressure to his own arm and note the time. Then, not looking at the watch, try to judge the three minutes that may be needed to stop capillary bleeding.

When the estimated three minutes is judged to have passed, check the watch. In all probability it will be very short of the full period.

Excessive capillary bleeding may be due to:
— coagulation defects
— capillary abnormality

Coagulation defects

The more obvious conditions which lead to faulty coagulation and which should be borne in mind, particularly when the patient is first seen at the consultation, are:

1. The patient is already on anti-coagulation therapy for some other condition.
2. Blood dyscrasias.
3. Vitamin C deficiency.

Capillary abnormality

When the muscle wall of the capillary does not contract, i.e. in Thrombocytopenic Purpura.

Heat

It seems illogical that heat with a hot pack will stop capillary bleeding when heat is applied to the skin by physiotherapists, in other conditions, to increase the blood flow and the circulation to one particular area. However, a hot pack can and does diminish capillary bleeding, probably by inducing spasm rather than any protein coagulation effect.

It is interesting that the author has tried sterile, ice-cold packs which work equally well, if not better, to control capillary oozing, but have the marked disadvantage of, in time, rendering the surgeon's hands completely anaesthetic from the cold which annuls the object of the exercise.

If a hot pack is needed, hot water must be provided by an assistant from an electric kettle and poured into a kidney dish or porringer on the trolley. The swab can be immersed in it, excess water squeezed out and then the pack used against the oozing area.

Visible vessels

Control of a vessel is necessary, either because:

1. The vessel has been cut.
2. A vessel is seen and is intact but is lying in the path of the incision.

If the vessel is cut and bleeding, the first thing to do is to apply pressure with a swab, not to go diving in with an artery forcep or haemostat immediately. The swab removes excess blood obscuring the bleeding site and by controlling the bleeding in the first instance with pressure, the vessel is given time to go into spasm and cut down the rate of bleeding. The cut end can then be visualised under control, and secured.

This is done by holding the haemostat in the right hand and then slowly moving the swab, held in the left hand, off the area where the vessel is being controlled until it is visualised and starts to bleed again. At this point the vessel end is picked up by the tip of the haemostat with as little surrounding tissue as possible.

This is an accurate definitive procedure and it is important that it should be so. If the bleeding is arrested by grabbing a great area of tissue with a haemostat, hoping that the vessel is amongst it, when this bulk of tissue has to be secured by a tie the local pressure by the tie on the vessel is diminished. There is also a mass of tissue which must become necrotic and have to be subsequently removed by phagocytes, which impairs the healing of the tissue in that area. The obvious risk of damage to surrounding vital structures included in the bulk tie is also a very real one.

Therefore, the vessel is picked up by the fine rounded end of the haemostat. This must then be secured by tying a ligature around it and as the first part of the knot of the ligature is tightened so the haemostat is slowly opened and then removed.

To get the ligature over the artery forcep, the latter should be held 'showing the tip', as illustrated (Figure 7.1). It is important to remember that this does not mean violently levering the handle of the haemostat and so stretching or tearing the vessel in the process. The tip of the artery forcep can quite easily develop a large lever action. If the haemostat is torn off the vessel the end of the vessel retracts into the tissue around it and becomes more difficult to find and isolate again.

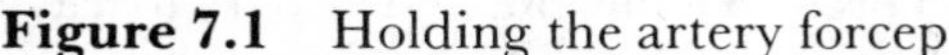

Figure 7.1 Holding the artery forcep

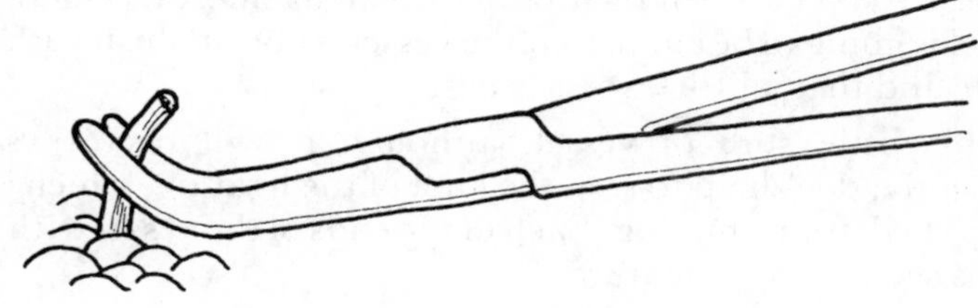

Knots and the method of tying them with instruments and by hand will be discussed in Chapter 10.

If the vessel is not cut but is visualised intact in the path of the incision it can be dealt with in two ways.

In both ways the vessel has to be dissected clean and clear of its surrounding tissue and this is best done by using a haemostat and putting the tip alongside the vessel and then opening the instrument in the longitudinal direction, so separating the surrounding tissue from the vessel.

This is repeated under the vessel. Whenever this is done the haemostat must be opened and then removed away from the dissection field before being closed. Only when closed should it be once again pushed into the area already freed and opened further again. If the haemostat, for instance, is put under the vessel and then opened to free it and not removed but closed in that position, there is a good chance that the posterior part of the vessel will get caught up in the anterior surface of the haemostat. If this happens and the instrument is then removed, the vessel is torn.

It is much safer and better to open the blades to clear the tissue a little at a time rather than trying to separate the tissue in one great wide division which tends to tear the vessel being isolated.

Once the vessel is dissected clean, it can then be secured either by clipping and tying or by under-running.

(i) Clipping each side with a haemostat and cutting the vessel between them. If this method is used, try and take the vessel accurately with the point of the haemostat, and also try to leave enough room between the tips of the two haemostats where the vessel is going to be cut so that the vessel is not cut flush with the blade and that a little excess is left.

This little stub of vessel, although it will necrose subsequently, does help to stop the knot of the ligature, which is to be applied, from slipping. Each of the ends of the vessel with the clip is secured by a ligature.

(ii) Under-running. Alternatively, once having cleaned and demonstrated the vessel it can be under-run by a ligature rather than being clipped. This ligature is then tied at the side of the vessel and the ends held, and the same manoeuvre repeated on the other side. The vessel is thereby held and secured by two ligatures before it is cut between them and then they, themselves, can be cut short, leaving each end of the vessel securely tied.

To keep the tissue clear and to leave a reasonable length of vessel to tie, it is sometimes useful to put the end of the blades of a dissecting forcep under the vessel.

The blades open naturally under their own spring and thereby open up the area freeing a valuable hand to pass and tie the ligature.

The ligature can be carried under the vessel by:

A haemostat being passed under the vessel and then being closed on the end of the ligature which is passed down to it, being held with some dissecting forceps.

When the haemostat is closed and pulled back with a ligature under the vessel, this has the same danger and fault as previously discussed, as sometimes the undersurface of the vessel is torn. To try to prevent this, rotate the haemostat a little so that the upper blade shields the undersurface of the vessel from being nipped as the blades close on the ligature just before it is pulled back, dragging the ligature under the vessel.

An aneurysm needle — Having cleared the vessel, the ligature required is threaded on an aneurysm needle with a relatively short length protruding. The aneurysm needle is then passed under the vessel. This is made easier by its curved shape.

Once under the vessel the short end of the ligature is held with dissecting forceps and the aneurysm needle withdrawn from under the vessel by sliding it along the ligature in the hole at its tip.

This ligature can then be tied round the vessel and when this is done and the ligature cut close to the knot, the aneurysm needle is left loaded to repeat the performance again further along the vessel. When it is tied again it can then be cut between the ties.

If working single-handed, it is much easier and safer to under-run a vessel with an aneurysm needle and to tie it in continuity and, having done so, to divide it, as it needs some practice for one person both to tie a ligature and remove the artery forcep at the same time.

Also it is easier to use an aneurysm needle at the bottom of a deep incision than to be trying to put two haemostats on and then to be tying them at the bottom in a very restricted space.

Principles of tissue healing and repair

A tissue defect can be due either to clean elective surgical assault with, one hopes, minimal associated tissue damage or be due to trauma with associated tissue devitalisation and loss. The difference between the two groups of injury is one of degree only.

In the elective cut in normal tissue the tissue on each side of the incision is sound and viable with a good blood supply, and there is minimal dead tissue for the body to remove before healing can take place. The amount of blood left in the space to form the initial fibrin clot is small.

Alternatively, in traumatic lesions there might be tissue loss from the trauma allied to the possibility that the edges of the cut are probably traumatised as well with areas of dead or ischaemic tissue. If not treated surgically these areas then separate later from the body at the line of demarcation and when eventually they have been removed the resultant gap that has to be filled and bridged, leaves a large area of granulation tissue and a large unsightly scar.

Also, if untreated and unexplored this type of wound may also have associated foreign bodies present which have all got to be shed or encased in fibrous tissue by the host's protective and healing process which, once again, delays healing and increases the amount of resultant fibrous tissue and scarring.

Whether the gap to be filled and healed is large or small the same histological process of tissue repair takes place.

In a connective tissue injury the blood filling the cavity of the wound forms a fibrin clot which rapidly becomes replaced by granulation tissue.

This is followed by capillary budding and fibroblast proliferation. The dead material is cleared away by large phagocytes and eventually collagen fibrils are formed and the granulation tissue is converted into fibrous tissue.

This process is very vascular and so the healing tissue at this stage is red. This vascular fibrous scar is later converted into an avascular scar of collagen which contracts and shrinks and, because it is avascular, it loses its redness and becomes white and pale.

At the same time as this process is taking place the epithlium at the end of the incision is thickening and starts to grow down as a sheet over the cut edges of the skin which, if separated and filled with granulation tissue, offer a bed for it to spread across to meet a similar sheet coming from the other side.

This conversion to consolidated scar tissue or collagen may take anything from three to 12 months. The time varies with the individual and also with the tissue being healed.

The degree of redness of any skin incision is a measure of the speed of this conversion of fibrous tissue to collagen tissue and, by inference, gives some indication of the rate of conversion of deep fibrous tissue to collagen tissue as well.

If this healing process 'overshoots' its normal, yet not fully understood control mechanism, then the hypertrophic or keloid scar arises.

In this situatiuon there is an excessive formation of granulation tissue and resultant fibrous tissue and eventual collagen. This causes very unsightly scars and is more prone to occur in pigmented skin, and in badly sited incisions going across lines of tension of prominence.

Fibrous and collagen tissue has no elasticity and healing cannot replace any specialised cells such as those found in the central nervous system or in specialised glandular organs and, in general, the greatest capacity for cell regeneration is that shown by areolar and fibrous tissue itself, and from epithelial cells from any epithelial surface irrespective of its cell type.

With this knowledge of wound repair, it is manifest that the resultant scarring and fibrosis of any surgical incision or trauma is directly related to the amount of gap that has to be healed when the operation is complete and so the tissues must be opposed accurately with their opposed surfaces being fully viable with good blood supply resulting in nominal debridgement that has to be carried out by the body itself.

The tensile strength in any incision gradually increases each day that the incision remains approximated with no stress trying to separate its edges. Thus, the use of supporting, absorbable stitches in deeply or stitches or straps for skin.

However, experimentally, the stress curve is as illustrated. If the incision is surgically opened and resutured half way along that curve, the stress curve of the new second-time incision is found to gain its strength much more rapidly and in a short while catches up the tensile strength which would have been expected if the incision had not been broken down. It has been suggested that this is due to the effect of a local healing hormone. (See Figure 7.2.)

This phenonemon is seen in surgical practice in such conditions as wound dehiscence with secondary suture where

Figure 7.2 Stress curve

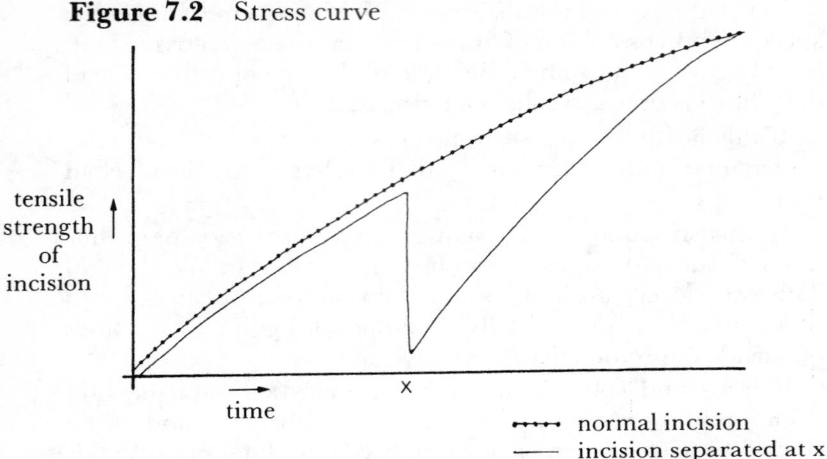

undoubtedly the secondary suture heals faster and stronger than the original primary suture.

Opposing forces can be due to outside extraneous tensions or internal muscle action but also, in the skin, can arise from the inherent elasticity of the skin trying to pull a wrongly sited incision open.

The direction of the incision in muscle, for instance, should be longitudinal — related to the muscle bundles. If the incision transects them, their inherent tone tries to pull the end of the cut apart while the fibrous tissue tries to be laid down to weld them together.

Thus, in both these instances, the tissue itself may be trying to pull the incision apart and so the siting and direction of the incision are vitally important if scarring is to be kept at a minimum.

In summary, for histological healing to be accurate and effective with little resultant scarring, there must be:

1. Minimal dead tissue that the phagocytes have to remove, resulting in tissue gaps.
2. No necessary foreign bodies that have to be removed by the phagocytes or subsequently extruded or of which the tissues have to enclose in fibrous tissue and which increases eventual scarring.

3. No infection which delays healing and because of the granulation tissue response to the invading organisms both delays and distorts and increases the final collagen scar.
4. The healing site must have edges or opposing surfaces with good blood supply.
5. There must be no tension trying to retract the surfaces whether that tension is inherent in the tissues or applied by external forces until the collagen formation is completed.

As seen later in discussion of surgical techniques, these pathological principles should always be adhered to as closely as possible.

CHAPTER 8

Skin Incision and Excision

Skin Incision

Use of the knife

Apart from the variation in size and shape of the blade, as already discussed, the knife can be held in two ways.

In the first (Figure 8.1), the handle is held firmly in the palm of the hand. The grip is firm and precise and the knife blade is visible to the operator all the time. This is the grip used for cutting skin, subcutaneous fat or other mass tissue.

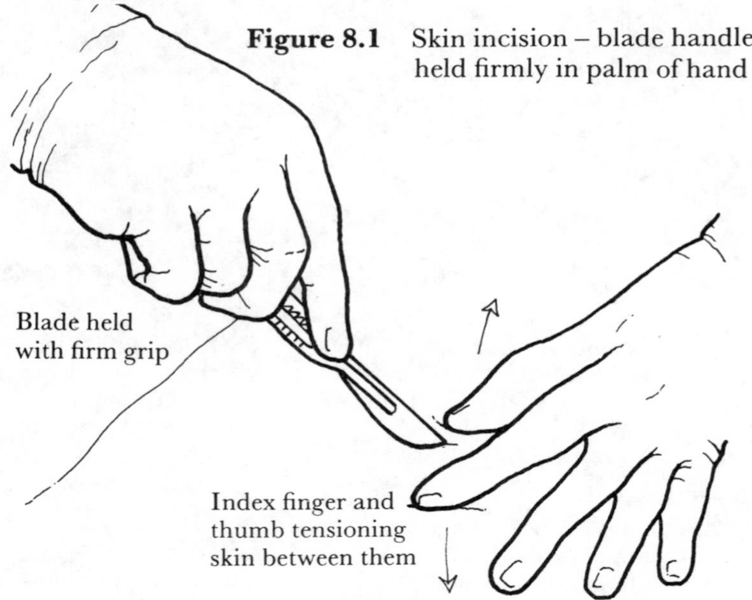

Figure 8.1 Skin incision – blade handle held firmly in palm of hand

With skin the knife blade has to go completely through the epidermis and dermis in one stroke if possible, and the incision must be at right-angles to the skin surface. This is so important that it bears repeating — the incision through the skin must not be slanting or oblique.

If the incision is not vertical, despite the most accurate of skin suturing, it is virtually impossible to get a hairline scar because of the inevitable, albeit small, loss of skin or distortion (Figure 8.2), thus resulting in a wide scar.

Figure 8.2 Non-vertical incision resulting in wide scar, as opposed to vertical incision resulting in linear scar

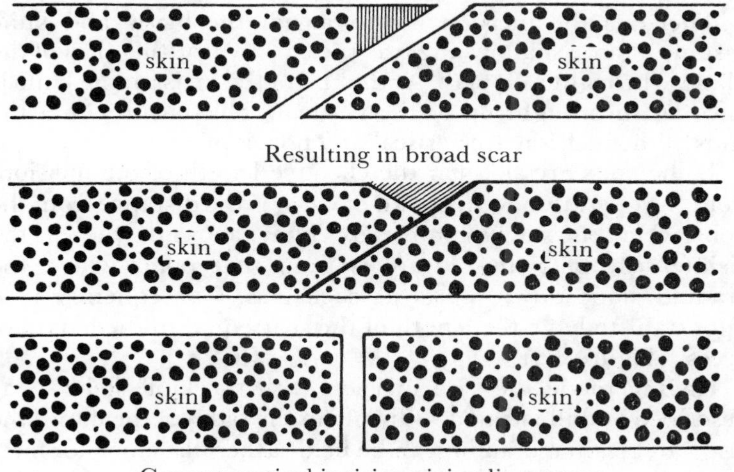

To facilitate the cut being vertical the blade must not only be held firmly but the head and eyes of the operator must be above the blade. Only if it is can the angle be judged accurately. Mistakes in the angulation of the blade surface against the skin are usually the result of wrong positioning of the head, rather than the hands.

To breach the skin leaving a smooth cut, the blade must be drawn against a stretched surface, otherwise the skin rucks up ahead of the blade causing hatching of the incision. Therefore, there must be tension put on the skin in the opposite direction to the direction of the blade movement and this is provided by the left hand (unless the blade is being held in the left hand to cut, when it is the right hand. This tension is best achieved by putting the thumb and index finger on each side of the proposed spot of the start of the incision. As the cut is made away from this spot, the fingers are gently spread apart to tension the skin at right angles to the blade and are also drawn against the line of the incision to provide the counter tension.

The initial breach of the skin between the finger and the thumb must be done with the sharp, pointed end of whichever design of blade is being used. This usually means that the knife is held more vertically at the start of the incision so that the point of the blade can be pushed through the skin.

Then, as the incision is prolonged, the blade and knife assume a more shallow angle as the effective cutting part of the blade is brought into play. At the end of the incision the knife is once again brought up to the vertical. This ensures that the ends of the incision are vertical and not sloping.

If the ends are sloping, the effective length of the incision, from the operative access point of view, is the distance from the point where the skin is completely cut at each end, whereas the visible scar following suture is from that point where the gradual slope down starts at each end. Consequently it is important to have the length of the scar equal to the length of access (Figure 8.3).

Having made the skin incision with the knife held — as described and illustrated — firmly in the palm of the hand, the grip can be altered and it can be held rather like a pen for finer dissection work. Holding the handle this way mitigates against firm, hard controlled entry but is very useful for finer, delicate work, especially with the small blade (Figure 8.4).

Siting the incision

Hiding the Incision

In a great number of cases, the approximate area of the proposed incision is pre-determined by the operation that is about to be performed.

If a lump is to be removed the incision has to be made over it to make easier its exposure.

Figure 8.3 Length of scar equalling length of access

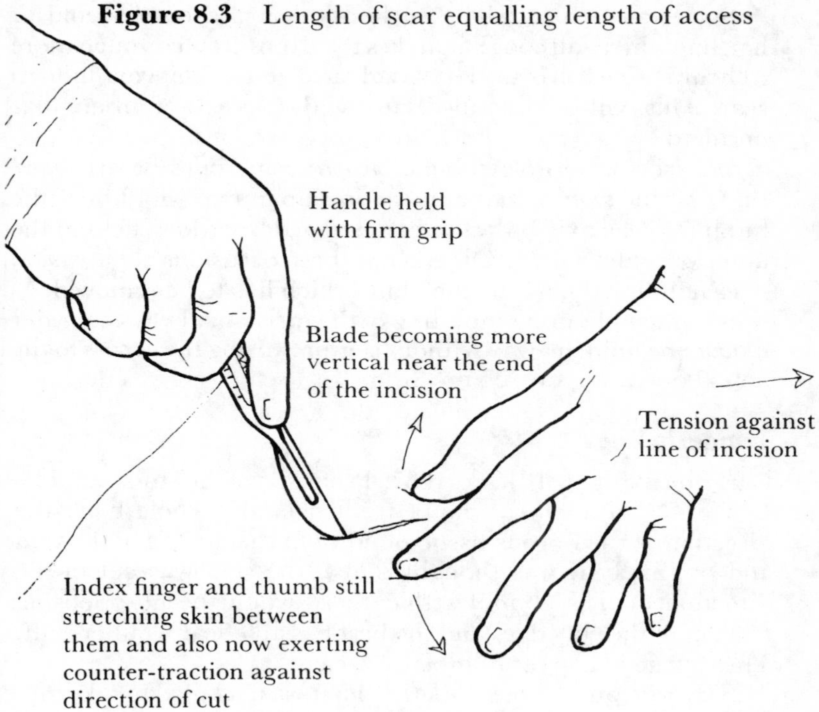

Handle held with firm grip

Blade becoming more vertical near the end of the incision

Tension against line of incision

Index finger and thumb still stretching skin between them and also now exerting counter-traction against direction of cut

Figure 8.4 Penholder grip of knife for fine dissection

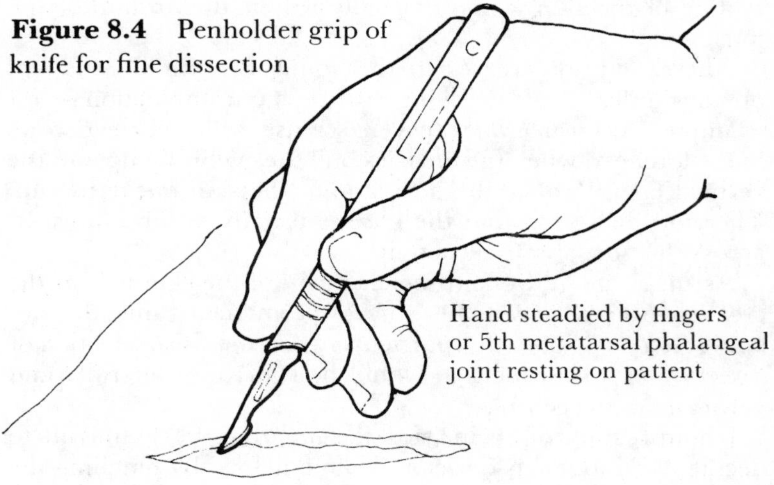

Hand steadied by fingers or 5th metatarsal phalangeal joint resting on patient

Sometimes an incision can be hidden in a natural fold or hairline which, although it makes the exposure that much more difficult, is well worth that disadvantage to achieve a hidden scar. This will be described later with excision of an angular dermoid.

With breast fibroadenomas, it can sometimes be arranged that the incision is made in the inframammary fold or if the lump is in the axillary tail it can perhaps be hidden behind the anterior axillary fold. On each of these occasions the incision does not directly overlie the lump which has to be removed.

So, when planning the siting of the incision, always consider if it can be hidden away without compromising the access to the actual operative site too much.

Langer's lines

Carl von Langer, 1819 to 1887, Professor of Anatomy at The University of Vienna, mapped out over the whole body the direction of the fibrous tissue bundles in the dermis of the skin and originally it was thought that if the skin was cut in the direction of these bundles that there would be no opposing tension to the cut edges and the best possible scar would result. This is true in a great number of areas.

However, admirable work though it was, it failed to take into account the natural elasticity of the skin and the movement and folding of the skin which normally results due to underlying muscle activity.

These folds or creases in the young are mobile and not obvious unless the underlying muscle is put into action — for example, the horizontal transverse creases above the eyebrows in the forehead when the muscles pull the eyebrows up and the vertical crease above the nose due to the skin puckering up. Therefore it is seen that the creases usually occur against or across this sort of muscle activity.

As the years go by and the elasticity of the skin is lost, the creases become gradually more permanent and do not straighten out. So, in this particular area, the site of election or direction of a skin incision would be transverse laterally and vertically in the centre.

The direction of an incision is sometimes very difficult to decide upon, but this decision is often helped by pinching the skin into a fold in a variety of different directions until the one is found where the tension appears to be the least and the incision can then be made at right angles to that direction. This should mean that the tension pulling the ends of the incision apart is maximal while the tension trying to pull the sides of the incision apart is minimal.

Although it is a little similar to closing the stable door after the horse has bolted, after a skin incision is made it can be readily verified if it has been made in the correct line. Although it does not help the particular patient in question, it should be mentally stored in one's memory bank of experience for future incisions in this particular site.

The two diagrams as illustrated (Figure 8.5) show the direction of the skin edges when the incision is correct and when it is out of true.

Figure 8.5 Direction of skin edges with correct and incorrect incisions

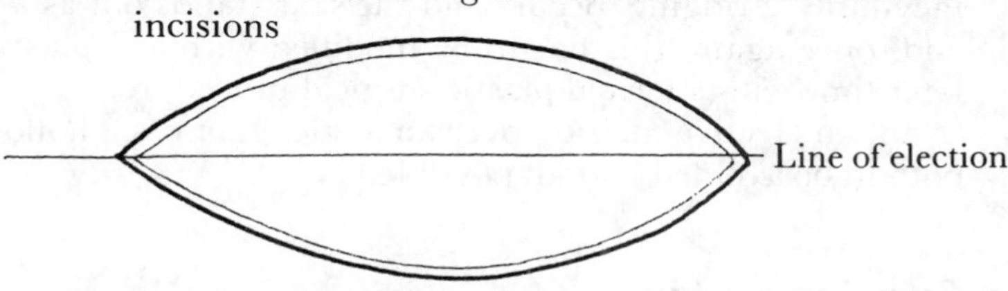

Ideal curves following excision of elipse of skin based along the line of election to give the best scar when the edges are sutured

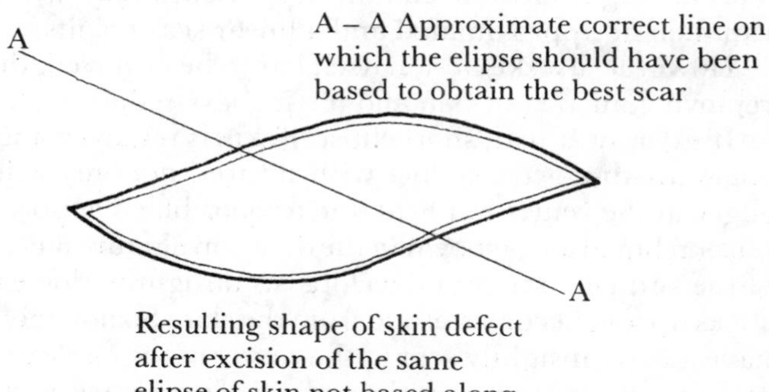

Resulting shape of skin defect after excision of the same elipse of skin not based along correct line of election

With the specific operations as described, the direction of choice of the incisions will be noted and in this way the total map of elective sites should be finally built up. These do not totally coincide with the original map as described by Langer, although the term 'Langer's Lines' is still used to describe the lines of election of incision.

A further basic principle of the siting of the incision is to never, under any circumstances, make an incision over a bony angle as this always results in a hideous, unsightly scar due to contraction. In particular think of the face with an incision going over the edge of the mandible from the face to the sub-mandibular region. A scar in that particular line which is normally traumatic, rather than caused by elective surgery, subsequently needs modification with a Z-plasty to get it at all cosmetically acceptable.

Incisions across a hollow also cause unsightly scars as inevitably 'bridging' occurs and the scar stands out as a ridge and, once again, this has to be modified with a Z-plasty at a later time with a formal plastic surgical procedure.

So, an elective incision over an angle or across a hollow are both to be avoided if at all possible.

Excision of skin

Up to date one has been discussing the incision of skin with minimum trauma in the correct direction to enable access to be gained to some underlying lesion that needs to be removed. This having been done and the deep tissues dealt with, the skin can then be approximated and a linear scar results.

However, if a skin lesion itself has to be removed, this entails removing an area of skin and having a skin defect left to close.

If a disc or broad, short elipse of skin is removed and the skin edges are dragged together with sutures, not only will the skin edges in the centre not heal due to poor blood supply from the tension but also, as shown in the diagram (Figure 8.6), each end of the suturing attempt develops an unsightly 'dog ear' which sticks up and becomes proud from the skin. So not only does one have a bad, unsightly scar in the centre of the circle or disc, but also protuberant areas at the end, all of which are obviously not acceptable.

Figure 8.6 Development of 'dog ear'

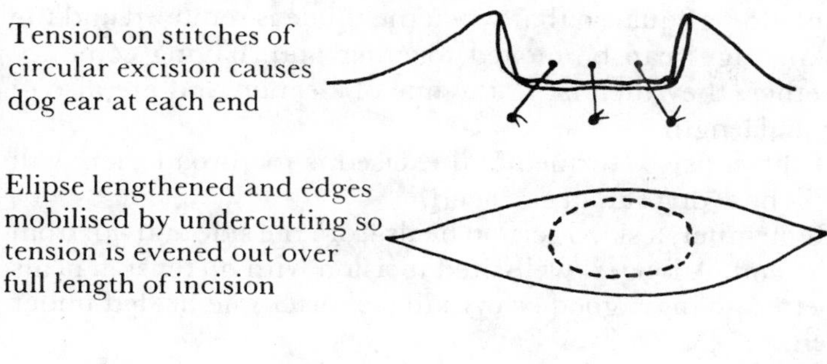

Scar longer but cosmetically better. No dog ears

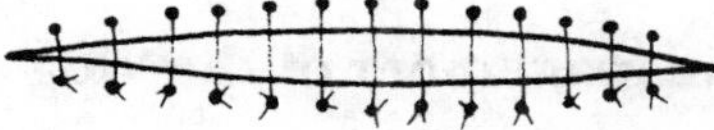

This immediately raises the point of the suitability of too extensive removal of skin being done under local anaesthetic as an out-patient procedure. If the skin closure cannot be carried out satisfactorily with a good scar, but needs some more plastic surgical procedure, then the case is perhaps more suitable to be done under general anaesthetic in a more formal surgical environment.

Thus, when an area of skin with a lesion on it has to be removed, to get a cosmetically good, final scar the following principles should be remembered:

1. To get a decent scar, the skin edges must be approximated without tension just as in the linear incision. To achieve this the edges of the skin may well have to be undermined in an appropriate plane to enable them to be mobilised and to lie loosely in apposition, so spreading the area of skin and 'borrowing' skin from a loose, redundant, nearby area.
2. The area of skin to be removed should be eliptical in shape. This elipse should be designed carefully with the following considerations:

(a) Having mapped out the elipse around the skin lesion to be excised, if a line is drawn joining the points of the elipse together, then that line should be lying in the line of election if it was only a linear incision that was going to be made. (Figure 8.5.)

(b) Having obtained the situation of the points at each end of the elipse, the length of the curve of the elipse of each side should be equal so that when the tissue is removed and the skin edges can be moved together and, having come together, they then lie in the line of election and are also of equal length.

(c) If the elipse so formed and excised is too broad there will still be a 'dog ear' at each end.

(d) Remember, a skin incision heals from the side and not from the end. A longer, well-sited incision with no tension heals better giving a good scar than a shorter one healed under tension.

The management of the 'dog ear'

The 'dog ear' is removed by a series of manoeuvres as shown in Figure 8.7.

The skin edges are first opposed with the help of any lateral mobilisation necessary to ensure that there is no tension needed to hold them together in place. The centre of the incision is then sutured and when this is done the full extent of the 'dog ear' at each end is demonstrated and becomes obvious. Having lifted up this 'dog ear' with a fine skin hook, the base is cut as shown in Line A. It is vitally important to get this cut through the skin going at right angles to the skin and not to cut the skin obliquely, which is the tendency, as the 'dog ear' is being lifted in an odd direction.

Also, it is important to take the incision right back to the apex of the fold which is formed by lifting the 'dog ear' up from the uncut skin at each end.

Having made this first incision, the redundant skin can then be laid over the other skin and the final cut made, once again taking care to ensure that it is at right angles through the skin. This cut is easier to ensure to be right-angled than the first cut.

The excess 'dog ear' is now exised and the suturing can be completed, resulting in a scar on a flat surface.

Figure 8.7 Removal of 'dog ear'

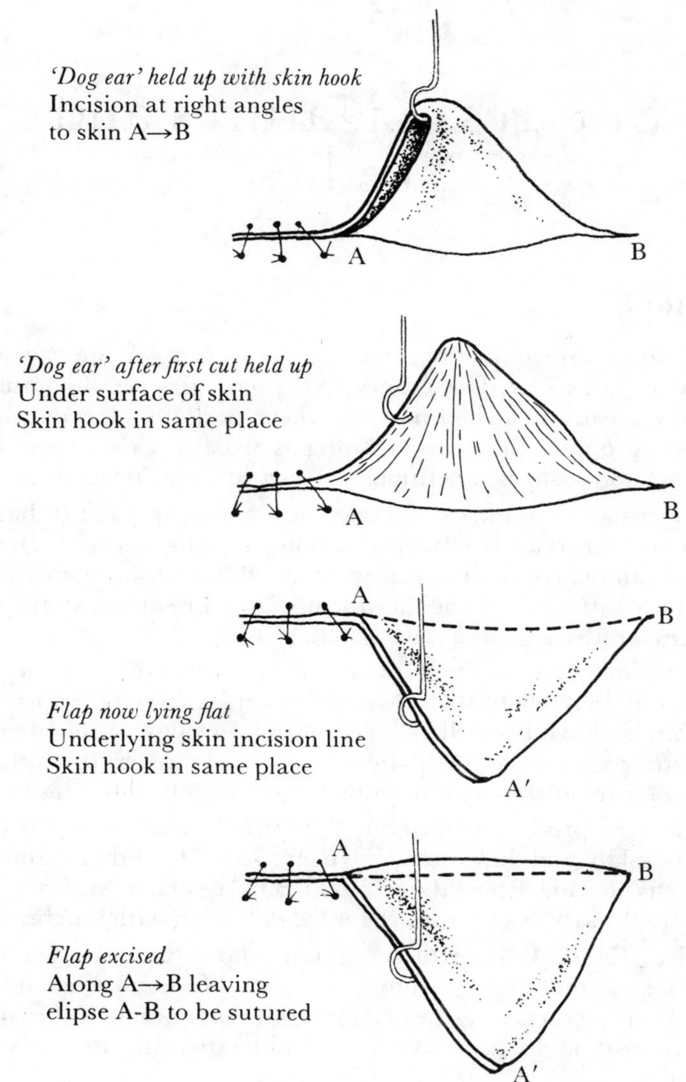

CHAPTER 9

Sutures, Ligatures and Needles

History

The word 'suture' has become a general term for the various pieces of 'string' used in surgery, in the sense that we often use it when we really mean ligatures. However, perhaps it is excusable on the grounds that the meaning is usually clear from the context and it saves repetition of the words 'and/or ligatures'.

Suturing of wounds is an ancient art and appears to have been performed fairly universally. The use of ligatures has been in and out of favour since it was invented, being supplemented by the cautery, at least for haemostasis to some extent, in patients under a general anaesthetic.

Eyed needles, made of bone and of a high quality, were available in 20,000 B.C. Neolithic skulls showing signs of trephining have been discovered with in-growth of new bone indicating survival of the patient. It is reasonable to think that some closure of skin was attempted.

Silk was produced in about 3,000 B.C., and strings from animal skin and intestines, even earlier. The Edwin Smith Papyrus, dating from about 1,600 B.C. refers to sutures — 'Thou shouldst draw together for him his gash with stitching'.

Circa 150 A.D. Galen of Pergamon, who sutured the severed tendons of gladiators, wrote in his 'De Methodo Medendi', 'Moreover, let ligatures be of a material that does not rot easily like those bought from Gaul and sold especially in the Via Sacra'.

This is believed to be a reference to linen thread. Galen continues, 'In many places under Roman rule you can obtain silk, especially in large cities where there are many wealthy women. If there is no such opportunity choose from the material where you are living the least putrescible, such as thin catgut, which quickly falls from the vessel'. He makes it clear in other passages that catgut was known many years previously.

Philip Syng Physick (1768–1837), an American who trained in Edinburgh, experimented with adhesive strips made from leather and noticed that they tended to dissolve after contact with fluid exuded from wounds.

Further experiments on animals with such materials as buckskin, parchment, varnished leather, tendon and catgut, proved successful in varying degrees and he began to appreciate the possibility of a suture which would disappear after its job was completed.

Joseph Lister (1827–1912), after much experimental work, realised that arterial ligatures of catgut were absorbed or replaced with host tissue. He eventually developed a catgut suture treated with olive oil and carbolic that could be stored in an aqueous solution. This was the 'carbolised suture' which soon became widely used.

Catgut is derived from the submucosa of sheeps' intestines and is over 99 per cent pure collagen. It is monofilament and is absorbed by enzymatic digestion by proteolytic enzymes from the lysozymes in Macrophages. Depending on whether the catgut has been chromatised or not, its tensile strength has diminished in between 15 and 30 days.

By the year 1900 the production of catgut on a commercial basis was firmly established in Germany, although originally it was intended for musical instrument strings. The word 'catgut' is believed to derive from 'kit strings' or 'kit gut', the kit being a type of fiddle used by teachers of dancing in the Middle Ages.

Modern Suture Materials

The size of all suture materials are now gauged in accordance with the European Pharmacopoeia specifications. This is a metric system using numbers from 0.1 to 8.0, each number representing the actual diameter of the strand expressed in tenths of a millimetre.

Sutures may be divided into two basic groups, absorbable and non-absorbable.

In general use today there are the following:

Absorbable sutures

Catgut As previously described, catgut is obtained from the submucosa of the sheep's intestine. It is a monofilament suture and is reduced to about half of its original tensile strength in seven to ten days. Catgut untreated, is designated Plain Catgut.

Chromic catgut This is so called because it is treated with a solution of chromic salts which has the effect of tanning or hardening the gut.

It also, with Chromic Catgut, increases its strength so that the tensile strength is reduced to half in between 15 and 20 days.

Polyglycolic acid fibres These are the newest group of absorbable sutures which are made chemically, being the homopolymer of glycolic acid or as a copolymer of glycolide and lactide.

The polymer loses its tensile strength in 15 days. The copolymer retains its own tensile strength up to about 30 days.

The extruded fine filaments of these chemicals are then braided to form a multifilament fibre suture.

Its knotting characteristics need special techniques and when pulling through tissue, due to its multifilament nature, it tends to 'saw' its way through.

These disadvantages, however, are being constantly improved as the surface of the suture is getting smoother as development continues and the knotting characteristics are gradually approaching those of catgut.

Non-absorbable sutures

These may be of naturally occurring fibres or synthetic filaments. All are treated to some degree to improve their performance or their acceptability in surgery.

The following are the materials in general use which would have application to the surgery envisaged.

Linen thread Made from long-staple flax fibres, twisted and treated with wax to minimise surface irregularities. This knots securely and gains in strength when wet.

Braided silk Pure silk, from which the natural gum (sericin) has been removed prior to braiding to ensure compactness of braid. Filaments retain natural elasticity, giving good knotting properties. It is usually proofed to minimise capillarity.

Monofilament polymide 6 Extruded single strand with smooth uniform surface which tends not to harbour bacterial infection. Knotting sometimes presents difficulties and a nylon type of knot has to be used.

Monofilament polypropylene Extruded single strand, exceptionally smooth, retains strength for long periods. More supple, it has better knotting properties than other monofilament materials due to ability to deform under pressure, giving greater friction and a flatter knot. Excites minimal tissue reaction.

Monofilament stainless steel wire Single strand, usually designed to have maximum flexibility to avoid tendency to kink. This is difficult to use and not recommended for minor surgery.

Braided steel wire Easier to use and tie than monofilament but can harbour infection. Also 'saws' its way through, widening the suture hole as it is pulled through. Not recommended for routine use.

Needles

Needles are manufactured in two overall design formats.

(a) An eyed needle.
With an eyed needle, where the suture material is threaded through the eye by the surgeon, the first part of the suture is double thickness so that the hole in the tissue has been made twice the size of the original hole created by the needle itself as it is pulled through.

(b) In the form of eyeless-needled sutures.
An atraumatic or eyeless needle has the suture material incorporated in the end of the shank and this means that the material itself is never wider than the bore of the needle itself. Thus, the hole in the tissue which the needle has pierced is always the same diameter as the needle.

There are variations based on these two principal design formats.

1. Difference in the type of body cross-section of the needle.
(a) Round bodied
(b) Cutting or triangular bodied
(c) Trocar pointed
2. Difference in shape.
(a) Straight
(b) Curved
(c) Half circle
3. Difference in size.
(a) Those to be hand held
(b) Those to be instrument held

Any permutation or combination of the above options are available and so before deciding which is likely to be the best, the characteristics will be explained.

Variation in body type

1. *Round bodied*

For use in soft tissue where the needle can separate tissue as it passes through it, i.e. in the fat or muscle.

Because of this it is usually the absorbable suture which is to be used deeply and is going to be left *in situ* that is mounted on this type of needle.

2. *Cutting or triangular bodied*

This needle progresses in cross-section from its point as a triangle with each angle thereof sharply honed as a cutting edge.

This needle cuts its way through tissue and is therefore used for structure such as skin or fibrous tissue in fibrous sheaths.

Usually, therefore, these are stitches that are going to be removed.

3. *Trocar pointed*

This needle has the part adjacent to the point in a triangular cross-section but very soon becomes round bodied, thus trying to gain the best of both worlds by being sharp to institute the breach of the tissue and being round bodied thereafter so as not to damage it further.

Variation in shape and size

1. *Straight* Usually stitches which are held by hand as opposed to those held in a needle holder. They are difficult to use in a deep cavity so are usually used either when the tissue to be sewn can be delivered above skin level or, in most cases, are used for skin sutures.
2. *Curved* This needle is shaped approximately as one third of the arc of a circle. Unless very large they are usually instrument-held and are usually used for skin sutures where fine stitches are needed.
3. *Half-circle* These needles ae shaped as half the arc of a circle and because of this are usually used in deep places with absorbable sutures where a sweep round with the instrument-held needle can contact rather inaccessible tissue.

Packaging

Today most suture materials are packaged in laminated foil sachets which are then overwrapped in a 'peel-apart' envelope of foil and/or plastic.

They are then sterilised by exposure to irradiation from radio-active Cobalt 60 at a dosage of 2.5 mega rads.

The synthetic absorbable sutures do not stand up to irradiation and are usually treated and sterilised with Ethylene Oxide.

Summary

As a minimum requirement, representatives of the following groups are needed:

1. Half-circle, round-bodied, atraumatic plain catgut, usually either 3.0 or 4.0 for suturing deep layers.
2. Curved, cutting, atraumatic with either fine nylon or mersilk for instrument-held skin sutures.
3. Straight, cutting, atraumatic with either fine nylon or mersilk for hand-held skin sutures.

CHAPTER 10

Stitchcraft and Knots

Stitchcraft

Principles

1. One way or another the tissues deep to the skin must be closed, so the dead space under the incision is obliterated.
2. The stitches, ideally, should be guiding and holding the edges in position relative to each other rather than pulling them together and holding them there under any degree of tension.
3. The edges of the skin incision must be of the same length, borrowing from one side, if necessary, (see later) to get a good scar.
4. The cut edge of the skin must be at right angles to get a good scar (see Incisions).
5. When approximated there must be no step on the flat surface between one edge and the other. Skin incision must be approximated accurately and not only in a longitudinal direction but in a superficial/deep direction.
6. The blood supply to the edge must not be impaired as this will lead to excessive scarring and delayed healing.
7. Skin stitches must be removed when their supportive role is complete. Removed too soon, the incision with any degree of stress either from the skin or from outside agents might cause it to gape and so give a wide scar due to secondary healing. Removed too late and the skin site itself becomes a scar due to epithelialisation of the entry and exit puncture holes which cause cosmetic problems.

Interrupted or continuous skin stitches

Stitches can be put in either as interrupted stitches where each stitch is tensioned and knotted individually or, alternatively, as a running or continuous stitch where the stitch is knotted at each end but the intervening stitches along the incision are continuous, i.e. the suturing material passing from one to the next.

With the one exception of the intracuticular stitch, which is a continuous stitch, interrupted stitches will be advocated for the majority of the work, the reasons for which are as follows:

1. They can be individually tensioned and placed.
2. If it is necessary to take some out early in order to try to get a better scar then this can be done leaving the rest in place under the right tension for perhaps a day or so longer.
3. If an infection post-operatively needs to be drained then one stitch can be removed without the whole incision becoming unstable.
4. A continuous stitch by its very nature cuts down the blood supply of the skin edge on one side or the other between each stitch due to the pressure which the continuous element exerts on that skin edge.

As the continuous stitches with the exception of the intracuticular stitch are not going to be used, they will not be described.

However, the intracuticular stitch (described later) gives a good scar, and particularly in a case where there is an apprehensive patient or a young patient, removing the stitch is very much easier and less traumatic, and for this reason its use is sometimes indicated.

The beginning and the end

If the wound to be sewn up has been made by an incision rather than an excision of skin, it is the custom sometimes to mark the skin before making the incision so that at the end of the operation these marks can be lined up to help with the accuracy of the suturing.

It is very much open to discussion whether someone who needs to mark the skin for a routine short incision should, in fact, be making the incision in the first place. However, if marks are needed they should never, repeat never, be made by the enthusiastic scratching across the intended line of incision with the back of the scalpel, as these scratches at the end may be the most visible and long lasting part of the whole procedure. If a mark must be made, it should be made with an indelible pencil, and there is a point in making the marks before the operation starts and the skin is sterilised.

With an incision through skin, by definition the edges on each side must be the same length. It is sometimes best to put the first stitch in the centre of the incision, thus making easier the equal spacing of the remaining stitches on each side.

If difficulty is found in judging the centre, then a skin hook placed in each end of the incision and pulled gently apart, will close the edges and help in siting it (Figure 10.1).

Figure 10.1 Placing a skin hook in each end of the incision

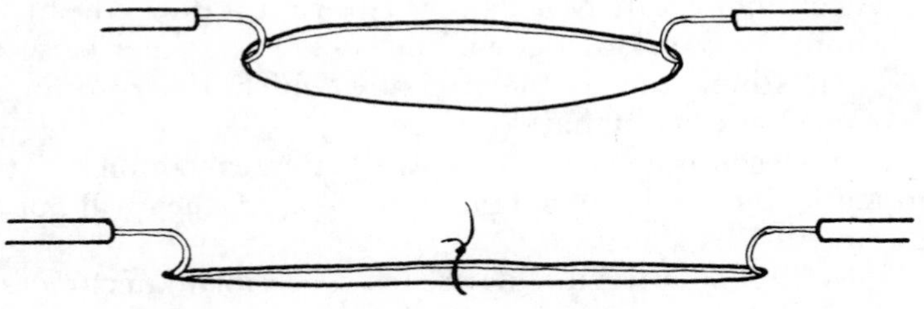

If there has been an excision of skin and the elipse has not been cut accurately making each side of an equal length, the one side will be longer than the other and each stitch has to 'borrow' a little from the long side.

By this is meant that whereas the stitches, for example, are placed 3 mm apart on the long side, they may be only 2 mm apart on the short side. Thus each stitch borrows a little rather than 10 stitches being 2mm apart on each side and at the end the long side having 10 mm of redundant skin.

In this situation, with differing lengths, it is very important to get the centre stitch in first, which means it must be at the centre of each of the individual long and short edges. Following this the quarter-length stitches can be put in. In this way the amount of borrow between the stitches becomes more and more obvious and also it becomes much easier to spread that borrow evenly — a little and often (Figure 10.2).

Figure 10.2 Spreading the stitches evenly

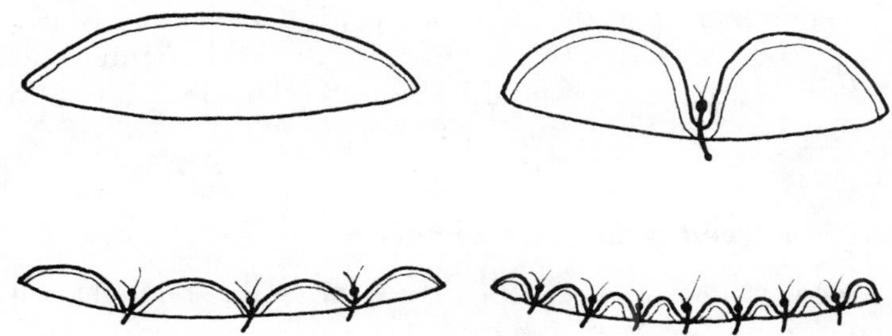

Tensioning of stitch

Just as scratches can cause quite hideous scars and can wreck the end result of a procedure, exactly the same problem can arise at the end of the operation due to the stitches themselves. The problem is not due to the siting of the stitches but is due to the tension under which they are placed.

It is obvious that the incision is placed in the best possible line of election to get a good scar. Therefore, it follows that the line of the stitch, just as the line of the scratch, which is at right angles to it, must be in the worse line of election for healing. If the stitch is tightened too much, pressure is exerted in that line of the stitch across the line of election, ischaemia occurs leading to scarring, and that scarring can be much more obvious than the actual scar of the incision. At its worse it gives a hideous 'step-ladder' scar.

The degree of tightening or tension in the stitch is a matter of experience, but the following points should always be borne in mind:

1. There should be no redundant wrinkles of skin apparent between the skin edge and the entry site on one side and the exit site on the other. These wrinkles imply that the stitch is tied too tight and is puckering up the skin unnecessarily.

2. There should be no whiteness underlying the skin stitch implying a loss of blood supply under the transverse part of the stitch.
3. The knot should be sited at one side or the other over the entry or the exit site, and not in the middle where it obscures what is happening to the actual incision.
4. Remember that the incision will get oedematous post-operatively, so as it swells a little it will tend to tighten itself. Because of this one should err on the slackness side rather than on the too-tight side.

Using a curved or half-circle needle

A curved or half-circle needle can be either round bodied for use when sewing up deep tissues, or can be trochar pointed or cutting edged when used to sew up the skin. These needles can, in fact, be large enough to be hand held, but this is not applicable to the surgery envisaged and so will not be discussed.

All the curved or half-circle needles to be used will be held by a needle holder, and the technique of using this sort of needle, whichever tissue it goes through, is a very special one.

Because of its shape, the point of these needles can be inserted under the tissue to be sewn at one angle and then, by rotating the needle held in the needle holder, the direction of the passage of the needle can be virtually altered by 90 degrees and further rotation brings it back through a total 180-degree turn so that it comes out parallel to its entry direction.

This is a very useful tool to have available for suturing deep tissue. On some occasions when instruments are being used to suture skin it is also, for the same reason, very useful as the essence of any skin stitch is to get the entry site and exit site at right angles to the skin.

The technique of using curved or half-circle needles is:

1. That the movement of insertion is a rotation movement;
2. That because the insertion is rotational and the needle is held by the needle holder at the shank, there can be a very big angulating strain of the needle at the point where the needle holder is holding it. Because of this angulating strain there is a danger that the needle will break;

3. That if the needle breaks, the major part of the needle then winds up totally buried in amongst the fat, or whatever tissue is being sewn up, and can present quite considerable difficulties in its retrieval;
4. That the technique of the rotation of the needle with the needle holder holding it at its shank, and the subsequent release of the shank and the picking up of the needle as it emerges through the tissue at its point, needs practice to acquire;
5. That having picked up the needle at this point it is then pulled through tissue to complete the stitch still in a rotation movement and not pulled straight out; it is the rotation movement of the use of these needles from start to finish that is important to remember.
6. The advantage of the needle of this shape is its ability to put a stitch in which, as near as possible, conforms to the principle of trying to get an equal block of tissue on all sides being sewn up.
7. One critical time is when the needle holder, which is grasping the needle round the shank, having been pushed and rotated through the tissue until the point of the needle emerges, has to be transferred to the point of the needle to continue the passage of the stitch. Whilst it is still on the shank, the point of the needle is grasped with forceps and has to be held there while the needle holder is removed from the shank and a new grip taken near the point.

Relief of tension

Tension must be minimised by undercutting and mobilisation of the tissue and/or skin. This mobilisation must be done sympathetically, remembering always that the more undercutting carried out, the more potential dead space is being created.

If an operative procedure has been removal of a block of tissue, i.e. an ellipse of skin and subcutaneous fat down to muscle, then, in order to oppose the sides of the fat deep down, it must be mobilised by opening up the plane between it and the muscle on each side with scissors.

This opening up the tissue plane is the same technique as described before by inserting the scissors, opening the blades, withdrawing the scissors with the blades open, then closing the blades and inserting the scissors again before further opening.

If the tissue which has been removed is only skin and the subcutaneous part has not been included in the block, the mobilisation layer is obviously much higher up and mobilisation must be carried out in the layer between the skin and the subcutaneous fat. There is no point or necessity in the latter case in mobilising deeper.

Once the tension is relieved, the deep tissues and skin edge will lie together naturally. The deep stitches are there to close off dead space and the future development of dead space being filled with oozing and the formation of a haematoma. The skin stitches are there to hold the position of the skin whilst healing takes place, after which they are removed.

The suturing of deep tissues

As has been said before, it is essential to get a good closure of the deep tissues as it is only by so doing that the surgeon can get a good closure of the skin and a resultant good scar. A good closure also very much diminishes the chance of any post-operative complication.

Deep fat or superficial fatty layers after mobilisation have to be closed so that there is no physical dead space left at the end of the operation, nor is there any potential dead space which oozing of blood can spread out to make way for a haematoma to develop.

This implies that the pressure that is going to be exerted on the deep tissues, as long as mobilisation has been carried out satisfactorily, is going to be the pressure exerted by the blood pressure oozing into the potential space, trying to open it out.

This, obviously, is a slightly naive description as any movement or stress on the part from outside agencies must be considered, but the point is made that the catgut stitches, which are needed to approximate the deep tissues, need be only fine plain catgut. There is no indication to use a thick plain catgut or chromic catgut to hold these tissues together, as it is totally unnecessary and also creates problems through delayed absorption.

The fatty layer, depending on its depth, can be closed by these individual stitches of plain catgut or, if the layer is just a superficial thin layer of fat, and not too deep, it may be more convenient to close this layer with the skin closure using one stitch such as the vertical mattress.

The fat is a poor medium to stitch as stitches do tend to pull through it and so, unless some fascial plane or some fascial tissue can be included with the fat, it is impossible to drag the fat together by tension on the stitches as the stitches themselves will cut through. As said before, the stitches must be a fine plain catgut because of absorption and also because the knot area, in particular with thicker gut, is sometimes refractory to absorption.

Deep fat stitches are best inserted with a curved or with a half circle needle. The needle should, on all occasions, be round bodied which will tend to push its way through the fat and, if it is pushed through alongside a vessel, will not cut it, whereas a cutting needle causes more bleeding by its own nature.

The essential thing to remember is that the movement for putting the stitch in the tissues is a circular one as near to rotation around the axis of the needle as possible. Not only is the needle put through the tissues in a rotary way, but when the needle holder is removed from the shank and put on near the tip to complete the passage of the needle, this action must still be in a rotary movement.

As illustrated (Figure 10.3) it is preferable for the needle point to be started deep on the first side and then rotated out under the skin following which it is then passed to the other side and is rotated through the fat, starting under the skin and rotating out deep. This means that the knot will be tied deep and as far away from the skin suture line as possible.

Usually end stitches can be put in this way round as the end stitches do still allow room for the knot to be tied deeply, and it is in these circumsances that those knots should be tied with an instrument.

However, it is obvious that the final one or two stitches closing off the fatty layer cannot be tied deeply and so these are put in in the reverse way, starting the stitch through the fat superficially and rotating it to come out deep, and then to the

Figure 10.3 Suturing deep tissue

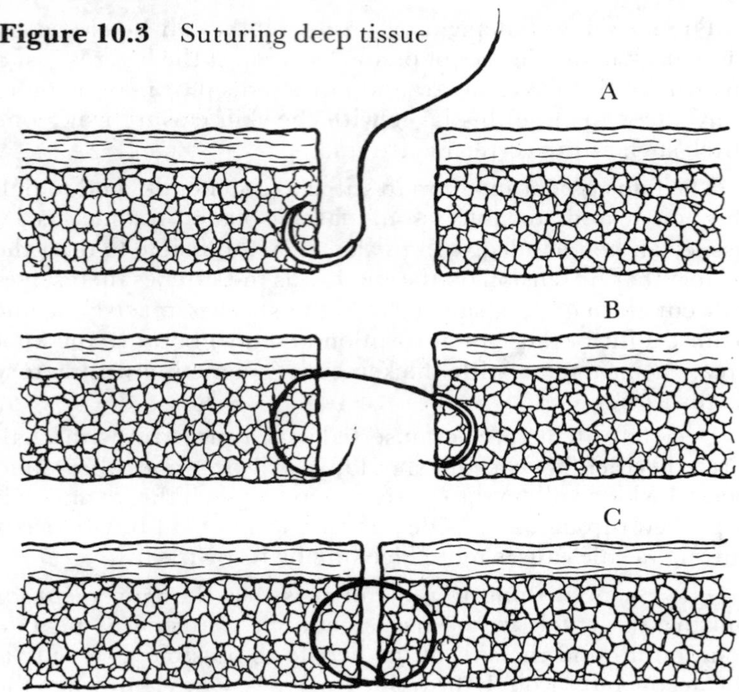

other side deep, rotating it to come out superficial, meaning that the knot will be tied superficially.

As many knots as can be kept buried as far away from the incision, the less likelihood there is of any post-operative problems with absorption and discharge.

Superficial skin apposition

The secret in getting good skin apposition is to get good, accurate deep-tissue apposition. This means that the skin edges should lie against each other without tension, as explained earlier. This skin apposition can be carried out by different methods or a combination of these methods.

1. *Simple through-and-through stitches* — to be described later.
2. *Intracuticular stitch* — to be described later.
3. *Straps* Straps or steristrip-type of skin closure are adhesive bands which are laid across the skin edge holding the sides in apposition. This is a method of closing the skin which it

holds in place whilst healing occurs but which, in fact, does not oppose any of the deeper structures. Straps are very useful in those cases where deep apposition of the deeper tissues has been very satisfactorily carried out, but are of more use in combination with skin stitches which will be described later.

4. *Clips* Silver or steel clips which are pressed over the skin edges to bring them together may be a quicker way to close a skin incision than inserting accurate stitches, but the very nature of the design of any clip implies that the blood supply is diminished in that area. Also the adjustment of the pressure is that much more difficult. They are very painful to have in, and are equally uncomfortable and painful when they are removed. It is considered that clips should not be included in the armamentarium of a surgeon doing the type of surgery envisaged here.
5. *Mattress stitches* If the deep tissue is not completely opposed up to the subcutaneous layer then the skin stitches, rather than being just through the skin, have to be deeper, incorporating some of the deep tissues with it. This stitch can be either an interrupted through-and-through stitch, or an interrupted vertical mattress stitch which will be described later.

Whichever type of stitch is used, the principles are always the same.

The interrupted through-and-through stitch

To repeat the principles that are being aimed at:

1. The entrance tract of the skin must be at right angles to the surface of the skin.
2. The exit tract must be at right angles to the surface of the skin.
3. The distance of the entry site from the skin edge must equal the depth of the skin through which the stitch is passing as shown below (Figure 10.4).

With a hand-held straight needle

The skin edge is grasped with either a Mayo or fine tissue forceps or, alternatively, is hooked with a very fine skin hook.

Figure 10.4 The interrupted through-and-through stitch

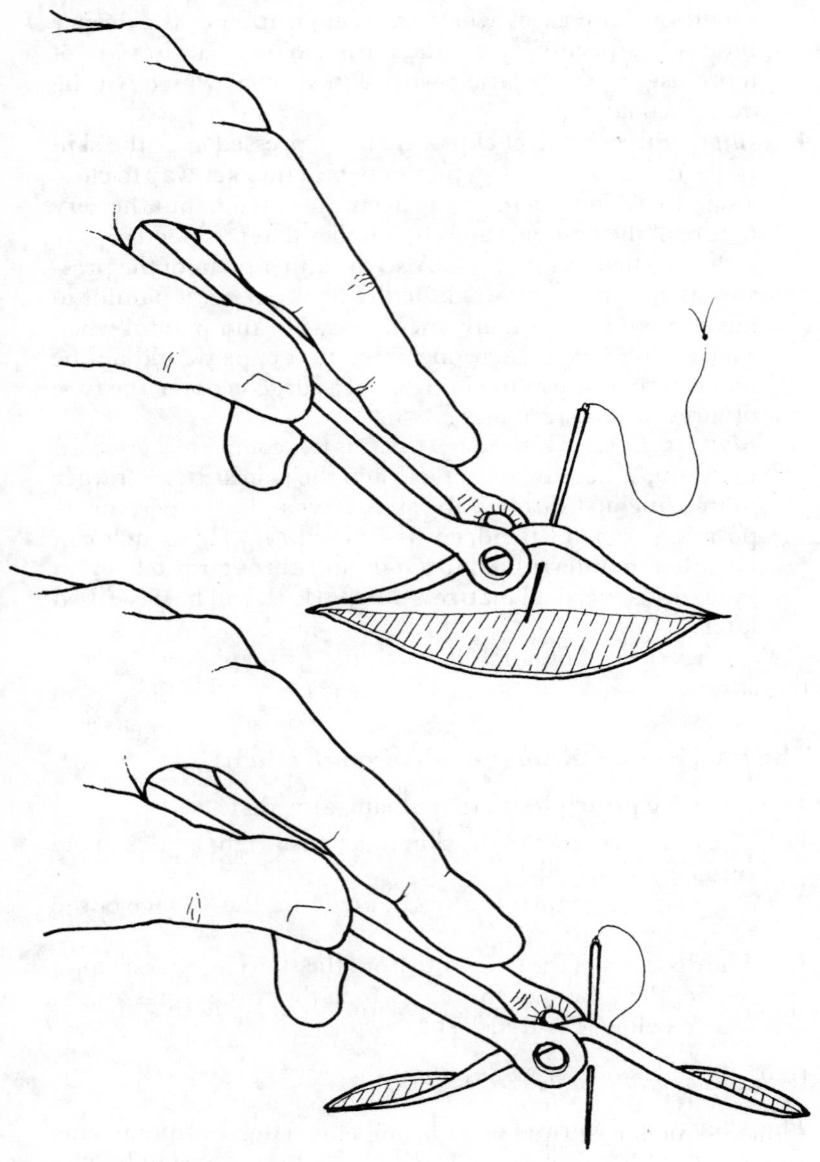

1. Using any of these instruments it is everted and turned so that its edge is facing out at right angles to the surface of the skin.
2. This enables the thickness of the skin to be judged.
3. The needle is then passed through the everted skin parallel with the patient's skin which, therefore, is at right angles to the everted edge, the entry site being the same distance away from the edge as the skin is thick.
4. Having passed the needle through this section of the incision, the needle is grasped by either the hand or the forceps and the stitch is pulled through that side of the skin incision before the other side is stitched. This is preferable to trying to take both sides in one fell swoop as it ensures a greater degree of accuracy.
5. The far side of the incision is likewise everted, and the needle passed through it as before from deep to superficial, coming out as far from the skin edge as the skin is thick. Because of the eversion of the skin when the needle is put in it comes out at a right angle through the skin.
6. The knot is tied, as explained later, being sited at one side or the other.

The verbal and illustration description of how to put in a simple through-and-through stitch seems uncomplicated, but despite this it is a very precise procedure and one which needs considerable practice.

With an instrument-held curved needle

The situation, entry and exit site are as before, as are the aims and objects of the end result. The advantage of using a curved needle is that used properly it can more easily ensure the passage of the tracts being at right angles, particularly with the exit site.

The method of use of the curved needle is just as has been described before, and it must be emphasised again that this is a curved movement of rotation around the axis of the needle.

It must also be pointed out that the skin is much thicker and denser tissue and, therefore, despite the fact that the needle is either a trochar pointed or a cutting edged needle, it may offer resistance to the stitch being put in. Under these circumstances it is sometimes much safer to grasp the needle half way along the body until the thickness of the skin has been traversed.

The advantage of this is that the strain on the shank region of the rotation movement is diminished and therefore the risk of fracturing the needle at that site is also diminished.

Mattress or vertical mattress suture

This is a stitch to use when the immediate subcutaneous tissue has not, or cannot, be closed, as a separate layer. It is a deeper stitch which can incorporate and so oppose this deeper layer.

It is also a very useful stitch in those cases where there is a problem with the skin edge, either where it tends to invert, or in those rather rare cases where the skin edge, following an excision, has a different thickness on each side. The stitch opposes the skin layer accurately with the skin surface on each side flat and level.

The danger with using a mattress stitch is usually one relating to its tensioning. There is no need for excessive tensioning just because it includes a deeper layer than the through-and-through stitch. If this does occur then the blood supply is interfered with and the scar becomes a bad one.

In summary, then, the features of a mattress stitch are:

1. That it incorporates more tissue deeply;
2. That it accurately opposes the skin edges whether of equal or differing thicknesses;
3. That it prevents inversion of the skin edges.

Technique

The same principles apply to the introduction of the mattress stitch as to the previous through-and-through stitch.

1. The tracts must be at right angles to the skin and because it is going deeper and involving subcutaneous fat, it is important that this right-angle path continues down in all layers and does not taper off the deeper it gets.
2. If the deep layer has been mobilised, the stitch can be put in with a straight needle as both the skin and the subcutaneous fat can be everted as one layer when the stitch is being put in and, therefore, with a straight needle it can go straight through all layers at right angles to the skin. If

there has been minimal mobilisation deep down, then the only way to get a right-angle tract through the subcutaneous tissue as well as through the skin, is to use a curved needle on a needle holder.

The stitch can, for descriptive purposes, be broken up into two elements, the lateral side and the medial.

The skin and subcutaneous tissue, which is being sewn up by the mattress stitch in one layer, is grasped by either Mayo or tooth forceps and everted. If this eversion can be taken to 90 degrees then a straight needle can go through the skin and subcutaneous tissue through this everted layer, which will mean that it will be going through the skin etc., at right angles.

The entry site for this stitch should be judged by the distance from the skin edge to the entry site being the same as the distance of the entry site to the point at which it comes out of the deep tissue.

Whilst the stitch is put through there, it is taken to the other side, which is grasped in a similar manner of all layers in one with the Mayo forceps, and that is everted. It is more difficult to get this stitch through at right angles than the previous one, but one way of helping this is to put the needle a bit further in than is necessary and then draw it back before passing it up to the surface to come out of the skin from deep to superficial.

The exit site must once again be as far from the skin edge as the depth of the skin and subcutaneous tissue combined.

When this part or lateral element of the mattress stitch is complete it can be seen that it is, in fact, a very large through-and-through stitch. The same principles have applied but because the stitch is that much deeper and has included subcutaneous tissue, it is sited more widely from the skin edge.

The inner or central element of the mattress stitch is now carried out. The skin edge on the side where the needle is situated is everted and the needle is introduced into the skin at approximately 2 mms from the skin edge. It then passes diagonally to come out half way through the thickness of the skin itself.

Assuming the skin thickness is the same on the other side, the skin edge is grasped and everted a little there, and the needle introduced into the skin edge half way through its depth and aimed diagonally to come out 2 mms from the skin edge on the surface.

When this knot, being completed, is tightened, it will be seen that the outer element is taking the strain and opposing the deep tissues, whereas the medial element is not pulling the skin together at all but is just holding the edges in place.

The knot is sited near and over the lateral entry site which makes the accurate tensioning of it and its subsequent removal very much easier.

If the skin edges are of different thicknesses then a judgement must be made, after having passed the stitch through the skin edge, as described on the first side, at the level at which it should enter the second side as the distance between the entry site in the cut surface and the surface of the skin must be the same on each side. If they are not a step develops which makes for a bad scar.

Using a curved needle

The same principles as previously described with a hand-held straight needle apply when using a curved needle. The advantage of using a curved needle is that the skin and subcutaeous tissue need not be everted to such an extent, and the 'block' type of pathway can still be obtained.

The danger of a curved needle on a needle holder is always that of trying to lever the needle through the tissues and, by so doing, it breaking at the shank where the needle holder is holding it.

It is important and worth repeating that with the mattress stitch, although the skin edge medial element has a stitch tract that goes obliquely diagonally through the skin, it is vitally important that the lateral element of the stitch does not do the same but goes through at right angles. Unless this happens there is a very great tendency for there to be an actual or potential space deep down in the wound that will accumulate haematoma and cause potential problems later on. (Figures 10.5 to 10.12.)

Intracuticular continuous stitch

This stitch is used in apprehensive patients and children as removal of the stitch is so much easier. With children, if possible, encourage them to pull it out themselves — it is very rewarding when they do.

Figure 10.5 Mattress or vertical mattress suture – straight needle

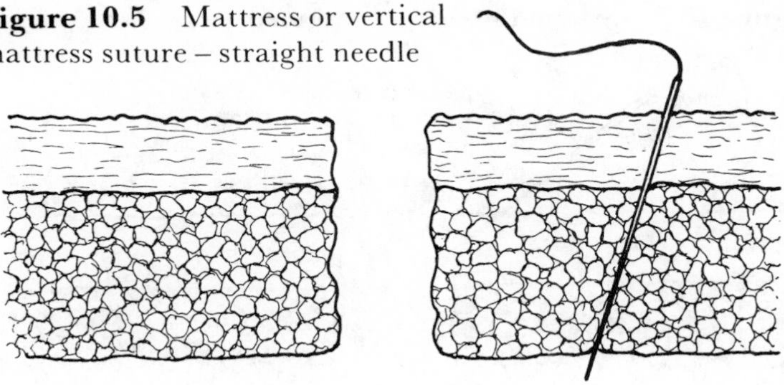

Figure 10.6 Straight needle – continued

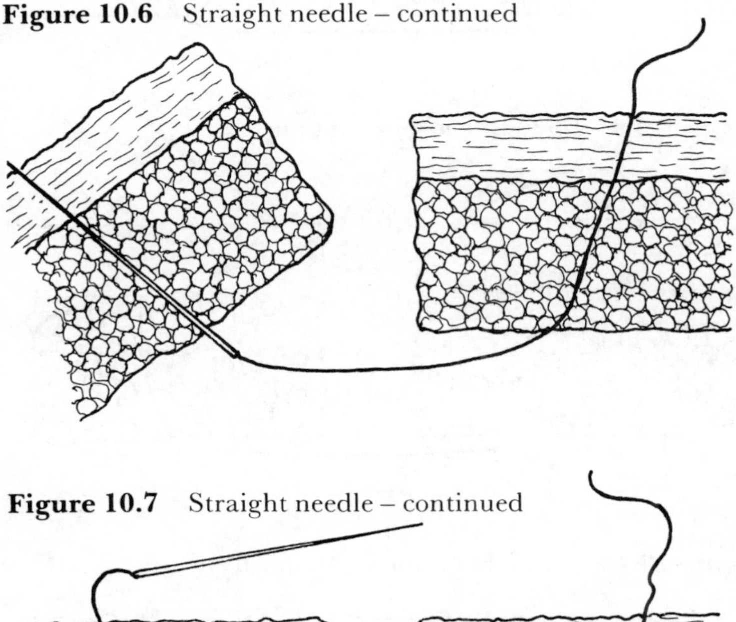

Figure 10.7 Straight needle – continued

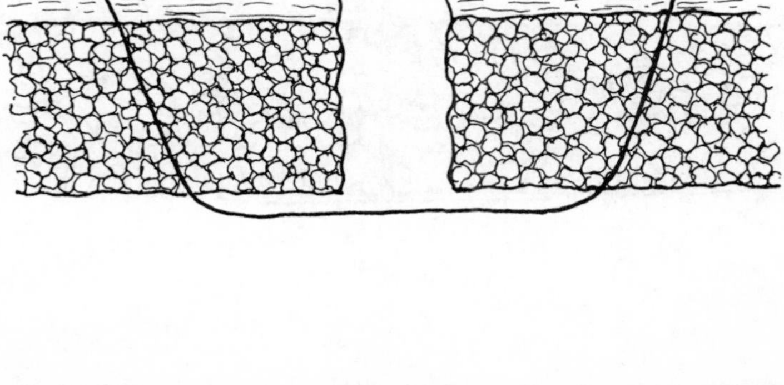

Figure 10.8 Straight needle – continued

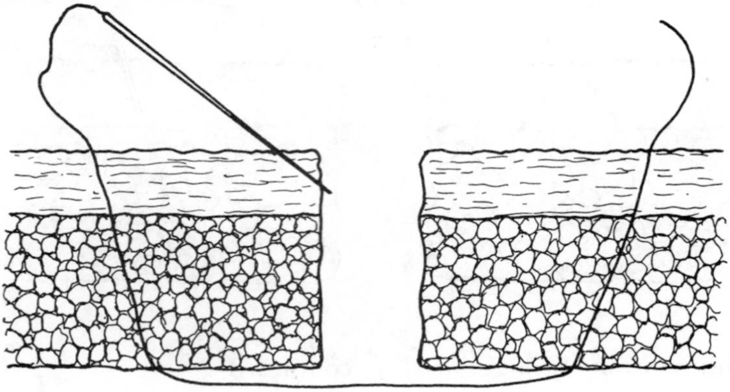

Figure 10.9 Straight needle – continued

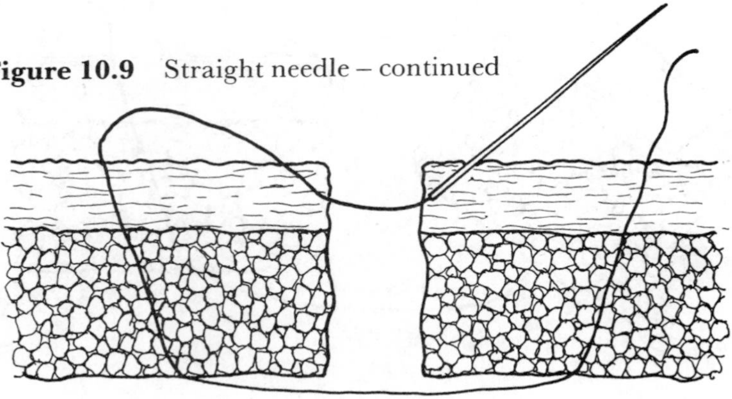

Figure 10.10 Straight needle – continued

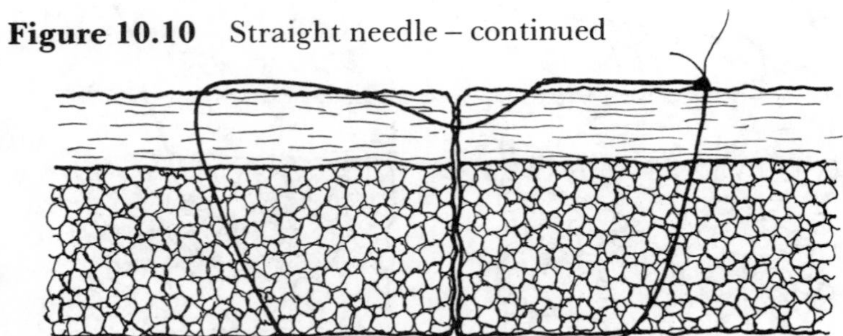

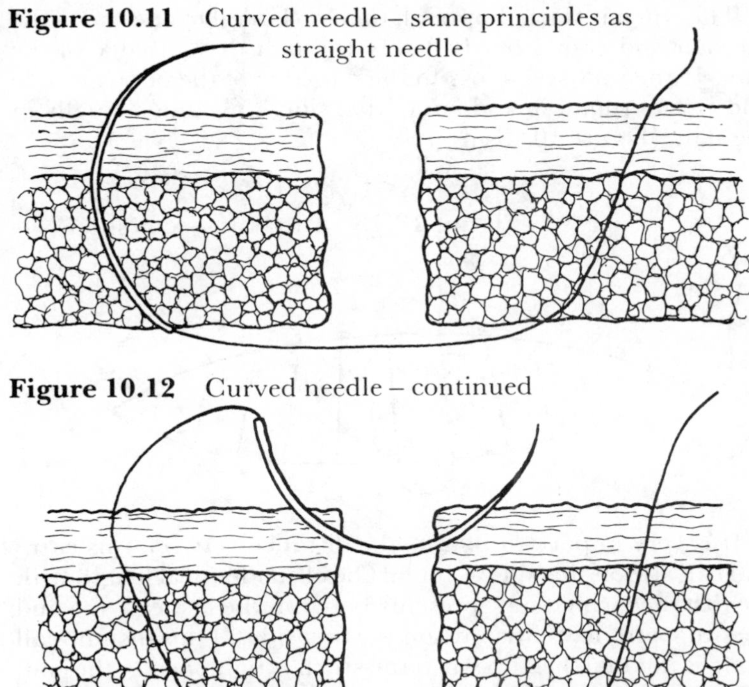

Figure 10.11 Curved needle – same principles as straight needle

Figure 10.12 Curved needle – continued

It is of paramount importance that deep closure is complete and satisfactorily carried out before this stitch is used as:

1. It is a fine skin closure stitch only.
2. A segment cannot be removed if deep trouble develops post-operatively. It is all or nothing.

Surgical technique

The stitch is totally intracutaneous, that is actually in the skin in its whole course. It lies parallel to the skin surface, half way between the deep and superficial surface of the skin.

It is put in with a small curved cutting atraumatic needle with fine nylon — never use any multifilament suture of any material. Nylon, being totally inert and smooth, is the ideal material for it and as there is minimal tension the very fine bore can be used.

The stitch is started through the skin lateral to one end of the incision and comes out half way through the cut edge of the skin. It then passes across to the cut edge of the opposite side and curves round in and out of that side, travelling actually in the skin. (Figure 10.13.)

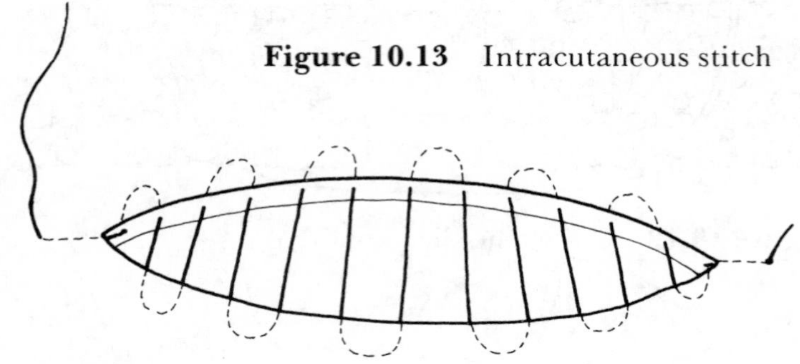

Figure 10.13 Intracutaneous stitch

It is very important to note the distance between this entry and exit site on this side as it must be of an identical length with the distance which now presents between the last exit site and the proposed new entry site on the first side. If this distance all along is not matched up when the stitch is tightened at the end, the skin surface crinkles.

At the end, the stitch is passed out through the skin to come out lateral to the lateral end of the incision. When this stitch is gently tightened by holding each end of the nylon and pulling, the two opposing edges of the skin come together and this is maintained by there being gentle traction on the stitch. The best way to hold this is to use what fishermen call a 'split lead shot'. This is lead shot which is partially divided, and is put over the nylon flush to the skin and then squeezed with a heavy duty Kocher artery forcep and, by so doing, it grips the nylon. The same procedure is carried out at the other end.

The nylon on the outside of the split shot on each side is cut leaving a length of about 5 or 8 cm. It is not cut flush with the lead shot.

Usually with a subcuticular stitch it is a good thing to apply Steristrip dressings as well across the incision. This means that when the stitch is taken out the Steristrip dressings are in place and need not be disturbed.

Removal of stitches

It is a very good practice, if at all possible, for the surgeon who has put in the stitches to be the one who removes them, rather than delegating this responsibility to a nurse or colleague. The reasons for this are:

1. A decision may have to be made whether all the stitches are removed, or only a few, and that can be made only by the person on the spot at the time the patient is presenting, and the person who makes the decision should be the surgeon who put the stitches in. So, if instead of removing all the stitches he feels for some reason or another that only alternate ones should be removed at that session and the rest removed at a later date, then that decision is his: it is a decision that would be impossible for anyone else to make.
2. If the stitches have been put in incorrectly, too tightly, etc., it is a salutary lesson for the surgeon who put them in and although it may not benefit the specific patient in question, it should improve his technique on subsequent occasions for other patients in the future.
3. Not only are the stitches examined, but the direction and siting of the incision is also examined and if this has been sited incorrectly and is obviously not going to give such a good cosmetic scar as it might have done, it will be remembered for the future. Just as important is that if it is sited correctly then that direction and positioning of the scar should be either mentally or physically documented for future use.
4. If everything has gone well it is a very good thing for the surgeon to have the final accolade of removing the stitches and maybe getting a round of applause from the patient. All of which can be no bad thing as far as doctor/patient relationships are concerned.

Removal of mattress or through-and-through stitch

Following cleaning the area with Savlon, the end of the stitch is grasped and lifted a little, showing the small area between knot and the skin.

This part of the stitch, as seen in Figure 10.14, is divided either with a knife blade or with fine-pointed scissors. It is important to pull the stitch out correctly and it should always

Figure 10.14 Removal of stitches

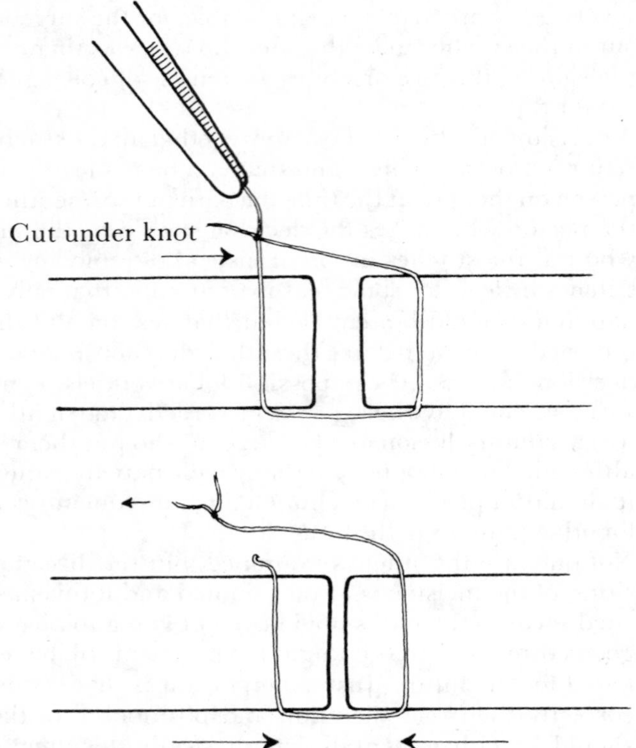

As the stitch is pulled out, the edges are pulled together

be remembered that it should be pulled out so that any stress being exerted on the incision by the stitch is always a stress that is tending to keep the incision closed rather than to open it up. Therefore, the stitch is pulled out over the incision.

Removal of a mattress stitch — this is the same principle once again of cutting the stitch on the lateral entry site as close to the skin as possible and then pulling the stitch so that the skin edges are tended to be pulled together — rather than being separated — by the stitch as it is being pulled out.

Removal of an intracuticular stitch

One end of the intracuticular stitch is divided between the entry site and the lead shot, the other end is then pulled out. With a child it is sometimes a good idea to encourage the child to gently pull the stitch out because it is painless and the stitch can then be placed in a small specimen bottle for him to take home and brag about to his friends.

If, by any mischance, the subcuticular stitch has been cut at both ends, or both ends have disappeared, all is not lost because a fine needle inserted between the skin edges can hook the stitch out in the middle. This is not easy, particularly with a child, and is only an emergency procedure.

Knots

A knot is a means by which two separate pieces of single or multifilament thread are secured together by a series of loops. This, when affected, holds firm despite any traction forces applied to try to separate the ends again.

With the knots to be described, in the context of their use, the two ends are of equal size and of the same material. This definition sounds a naïve one, but it is, nevertheless, a baseline to work upon as the type of knot is, in some way, predetermined by:

1. The type of material that is being knotted;
2. Whether there is any opposing force trying to separate the ends while the knot is being tied and completed;
3. Whether one end is fixed and unable to be used in the looping process;
4. Whether the knot is being tied with the fingers or by an instrument.

Type of material

The easiest material to use is:

1. One which has no inherent elasticity of its own and so is not all the time trying to spring open and uncoil and become loose;
2. One which has an irregular surface, which helps to hold it and diminishes slipping, rather than a smooth one;

3. One which is strong, which means that the same tensile strength of the suture is obtained with a much thinner strand, which once again gives a more secure knot;
4. One that, if the material is going to be removed when healing is underway, — such as in a skin stitch — must excite the minimal tissue reaction while it is present, to minimise scarring;
5. One where, if the material is to be absorbed, the thickness of the strand is important as the knot is where the bulk of the tie is concentrated and it is this that is probably the last part to absorb.

The problems

When tying up a Christmas parcel with string, if it is under tension, the help of another member of the family is sought to apply pressure with a well placed finger on the first part of the knot, to stop it slipping, whilst the second part is carried out and the knot is completed.

This is not a practical proposition while operating, so, if by mischance there is resistance to the tying — which, it must be said, should not be the case — then a different knot is used which may not be ideal because it may not 'lie right' and be bulky. This will be described in a special section.

Whether one end of the suture is fixed

One end of the suture to be tied may be 'fixed' by which is meant that it cannot be used to be pulled through any loops of the knot as it is formed. This usually happens where there is a needle threaded, or an atraumatic needle attached at one end of the suture, or where there is a much longer length of suture material at one end of the knot being tied than at the other.

Obviously in these situations the method of tying the knot has to be one where all the work is done with one end whilst the other end is held constantly in the hand.

Whether the knot is being tied with an instrument or by the fingers directly

Sometimes, if the access to the area where the knot is to be tied is limited, then it becomes mandatory to use a needle holder or artery forceps to grasp the end of the suture and secure the knot because the finger might be too bulky to get down to it.

With this exception, the choice of whether to use instruments or fingers is one of personal selection and usually boils down to convenience of use.

If the surgeon has been holding a large needle in the hand then it is natural to tie the knot with the fingers. If the needle is small and held by a needle holder it seems natural to continue, after the stitch has been inserted, to tie the knot with the instrument.

If a vessel is being tied around a haemostat it depends on its site and access as to which is the most convenient. In any case, the surgeon's repertoire must contain the ability to carry out both techniques. The basic knots and the method of tying will now be discussed and, subsequently, modifications for special situations.

The objective in tying a knot

A reef knot is the simplest and overall soundest knot to be used for the standard material described before. The reef knot finishes up when tied as shown below (Figure 10.15).

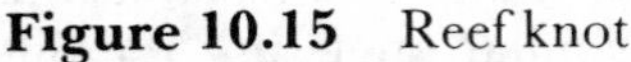

Figure 10.15 Reef knot

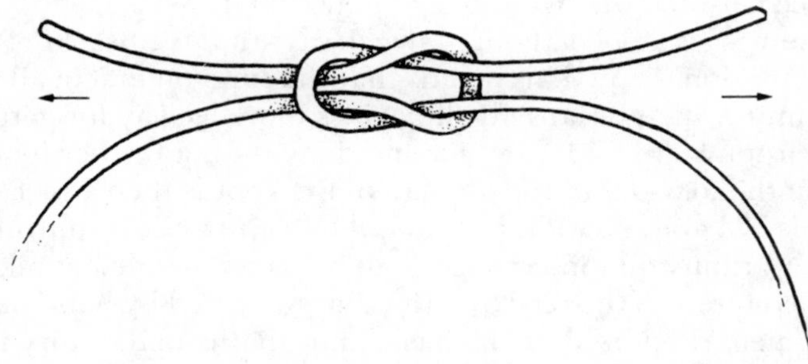

Reef knot

Careful study of this simple end result will show that the two loops, when so tied, tighten up and lock onto each other as any tension is applied in the direction of the arrows which is trying to undo the knot.

Note very carefully the difference between the reef knot (previous page) and the granny knot (Figure 10.16), which is not secure.

Figure 10.16 Granny knot

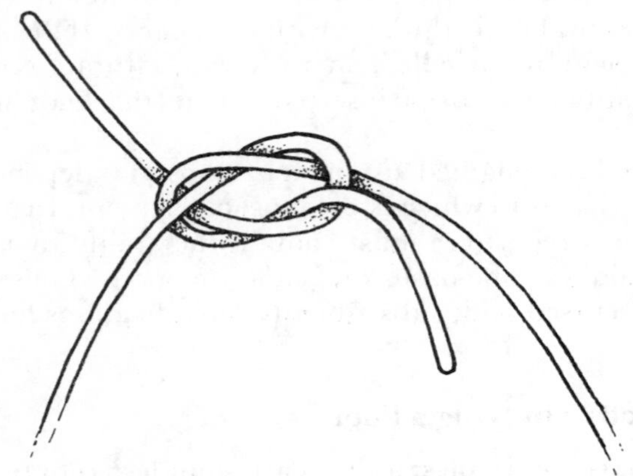

Granny knot

In the granny knot there are not two loops which self tighten with tension, so this knot is not secure and will loosen and slip. As can be seen these are two very similar knots but the difference between the two is one of potential disaster.

There is a school of thought which says that the best knot is a 'combination' knot. This means that the surgeon first of all ties a granny, which because it slips gives more leeway for getting the tension right and then, having done that, a further loop is put on the top so that the top half of the knot is then a reef.

This is a clumsy knot, bulky, still liable to fault by putting a further granny on top, and is not to be recommended at all.

Therefore it is the reef knot that has to be tied by hand or by instrument, and used as the basic knot that is mandatory in a surgeon's repertoire. It has to be tied with one end anchored and held or fixed, and it will be tied using either:

(a) an instrument held in the other hand;

(b) fingers of the other hand.

The importance of tightening the knot will be discussed later.

Tying with an instrument

The stitch has been put in place and on one end is a needle: it is this end which is called the fixed end, and the other, the free end.

The stitch is pulled through from the fixed end until most of the excess ligature is at that end and there is only approximately 5cms left protruding through the skin at the free end.

1. The fixed end is held in the left hand and all the slack taken up (Figure 10.17).

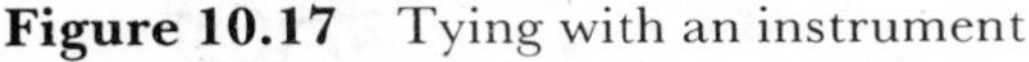

Figure 10.17 Tying with an instrument

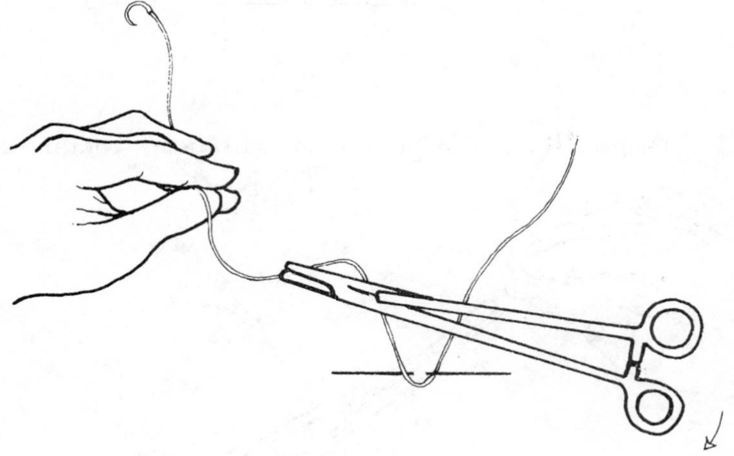

2. The needle holder is in the right hand and with the jaws closed to minimise snagging. It is looped around the fixed end by going on top of the suture to start and then looping behind it and under it, all the time with the jaws pointing upwards towards the left hand (Figures 10.18 and 10.19).

While this movement is happening, the needle holder is automatically starting to rotate in a clockwise direction, which points the jaws away from the left hand and towards the free end of the suture on the right-hand side.

Figure 10.18 Tying with an instrument – continued

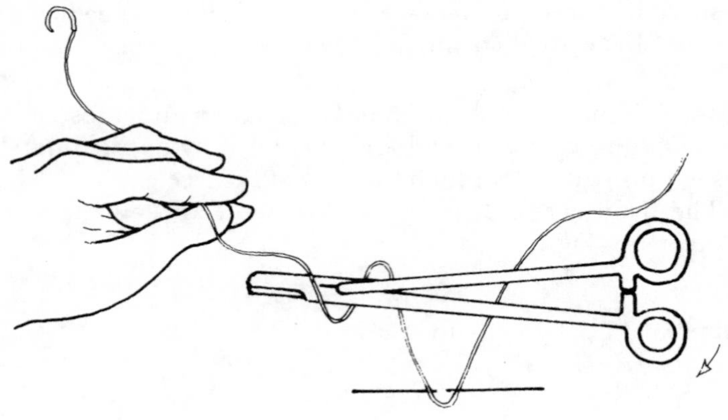

Figure 10.19 Tying with an instrument – continued

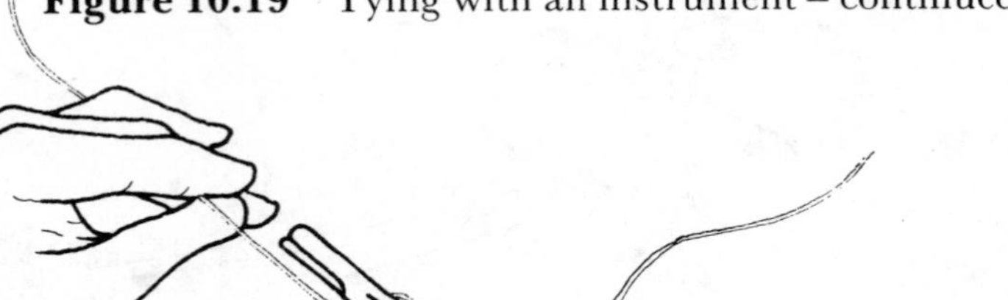

The jaws of the needle holder are now opened and the free end of the suture is grasped. The needle holder in the right hand is pulled to the left, and the fixed end in the left hand is moved over to the right and tightened against the counter force applied by the needle holder.

The first movement to complete the first half of the reef knot is now complete (Figures 10.20 to 10.22).

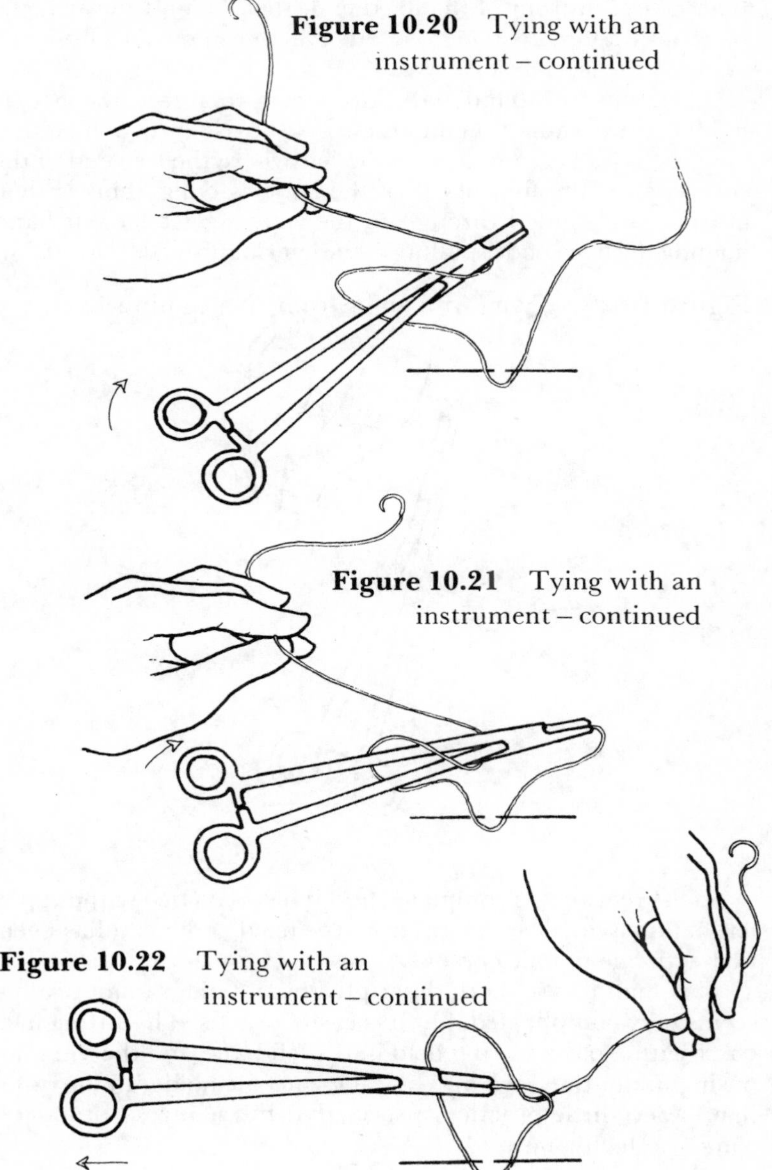

Figure 10.20 Tying with an instrument – continued

Figure 10.21 Tying with an instrument – continued

Figure 10.22 Tying with an instrument – continued

The needle holder's grip on the free end is now released and it moves once again to the fixed end where the needle holder is placed first in front of the fixed end, then behind towards the back and again to the front, all the time pointing upwards towards the left hand.

This time the hand naturally starts to rotate the needle holder at the same time in an anti-clockwise direction so that now the jaws begin to face to the left where the free end of the suture, after the first phase of the knot, is lying. This is then grasped and pulled through to the right whilst the left hand holding the fixed end is pulling to the left (Figures 10.23 to 10.26).

Figure 10.23 Tying with an instrument – continued

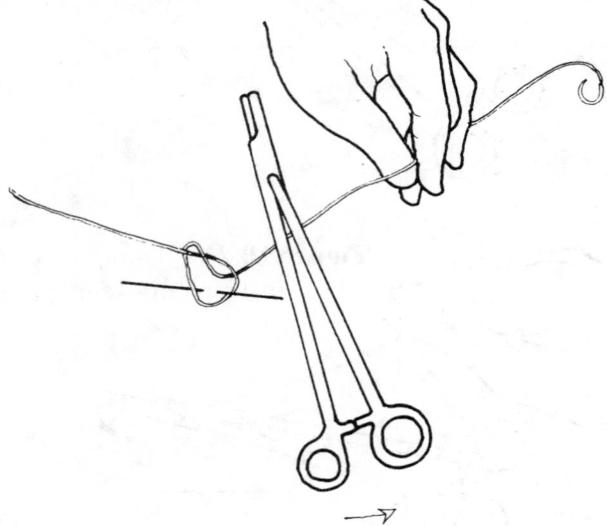

So the reef knot is completed and it has been tied without the left hand having lost its grip from the fixed end, i.e. it has been tied with one mobile end only.

This manoeuvre, both descriptively and diagrammatically, seems very complicated, but it is easily practised by sitting in a chair with a ball of string held in the left hand and the free end pasing under the thigh and holding a needle holder in the right hand. Very little practice ensures that the sequence of moves comes perfectly naturally.

It is vital to practise as if the second move is done upside down the end result is a granny, or an unstable knot.

The actual method of tightening the knot will be discussed later.

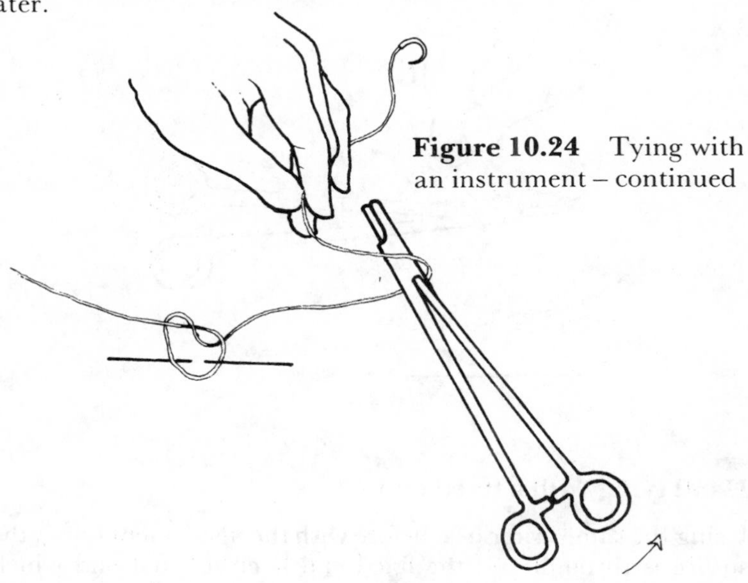

Figure 10.24 Tying with an instrument – continued

Figure 10.25 Tying with an instrument – continued

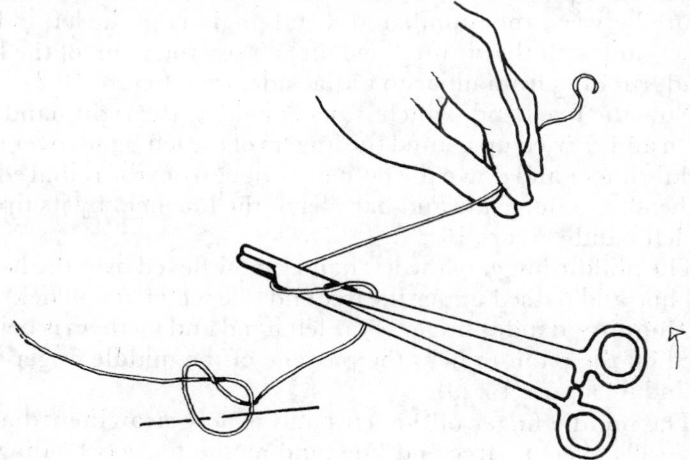

Figure 10.26 Tying with an instrument – continued

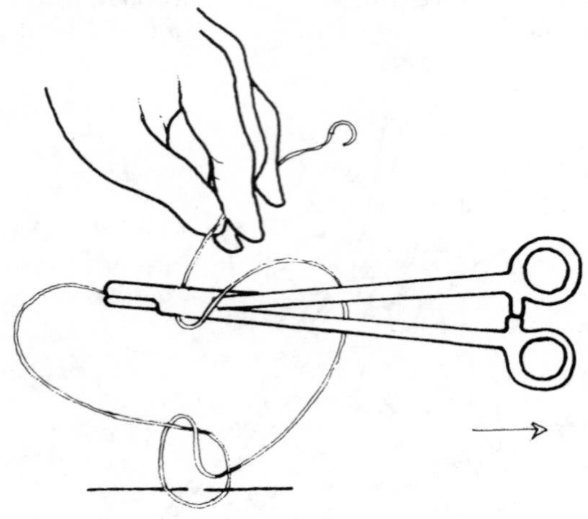

Hand tying with a fixed end

Using the same criteria as before with the instrument tying, the suture is through and the fixed end is either that end which contains the needle or, if it is an ordinary tie, it is the long end or the 'fixed' end which is held in the right hand.

The first position is to hold the end of the free end of the suture between the thumb and distal phalanx of the left index finger and with the suture line lying across the palm of the left hand, running from ulnar to radial side. (See Figure 10.27.)

Now the fixed end, which is being held in the right hand, is taken and carried up behind the fingers of the left hand, over the middle finger and down the palmar surface from the radial edge to the ulnar, alongside and parallel to the line held by its tip in the left hand (Figure 10.28).

The middle finger of the left hand is now flexed over the fixed end line and passed under the free end line which is still held by the thumb and index finger of the left hand and by them is being lifted off the palm to help the passage of the middle finger-tip behind it (Figure 10.29).

The middle finger of the left hand is now straightened and this pulls over the free end line, and as the tension holding it

Figure 10.27 Hand tying with a fixed end

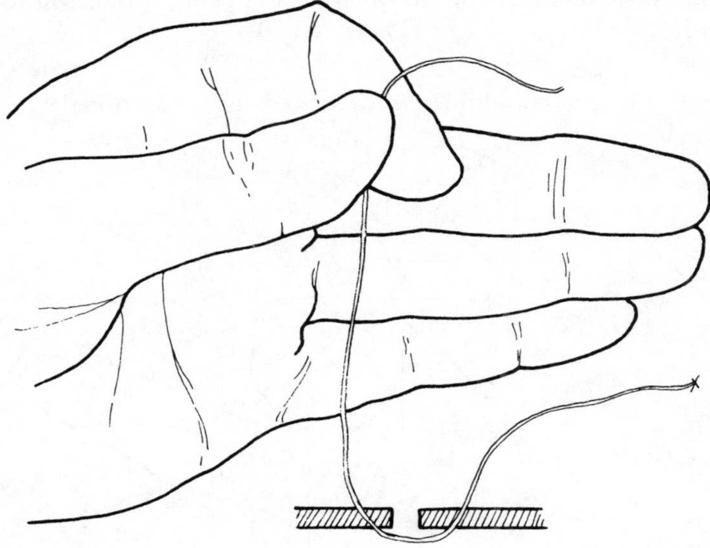

Figure 10.28 Hand tying with a fixed end – continued

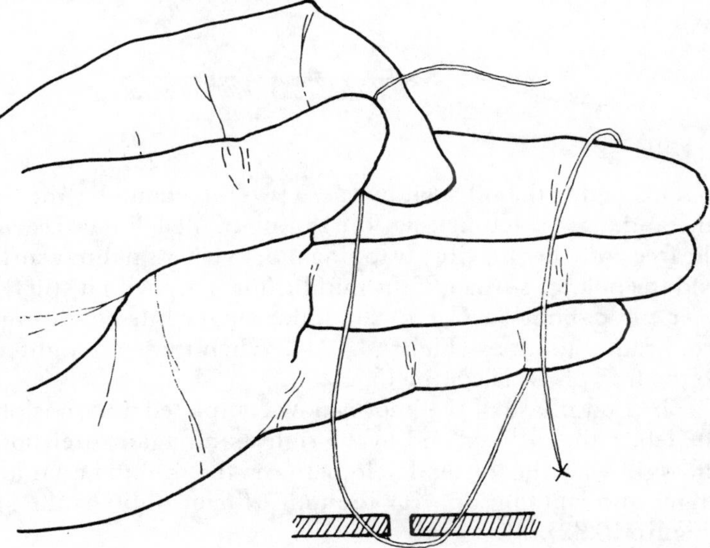

between the thumb and the index finger is released, it is replaced by it being held between the opposing surfaces of the middle and the ring finger (Figure 10.30).

Figure 10.29 Hand tying with a fixed end – continued

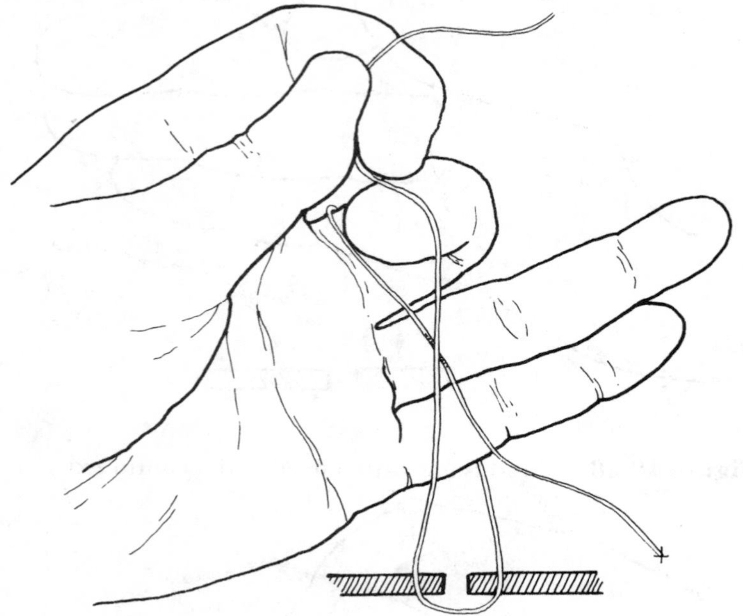

This end is then drawn by these two fingers under the fixed line and, as it is happening, the thumb of the left hand secures the free end line this time trapping it between its palmar surface and the palmar surface of the middle finger-tip with it still lying over the palmar surface of the index finger but now running from radial to ulnar (Figure 10.31). When these are tightened so the first phase is complete.

The first phase of the knot is now completed and tension to the left with the fixed end in the right hand against tension to the right with the free end held between the thumb and middle finger and running up over the index finger tightens the knot (Figure 10.32).

Figure 10.30 Hand tying with a fixed end – continued

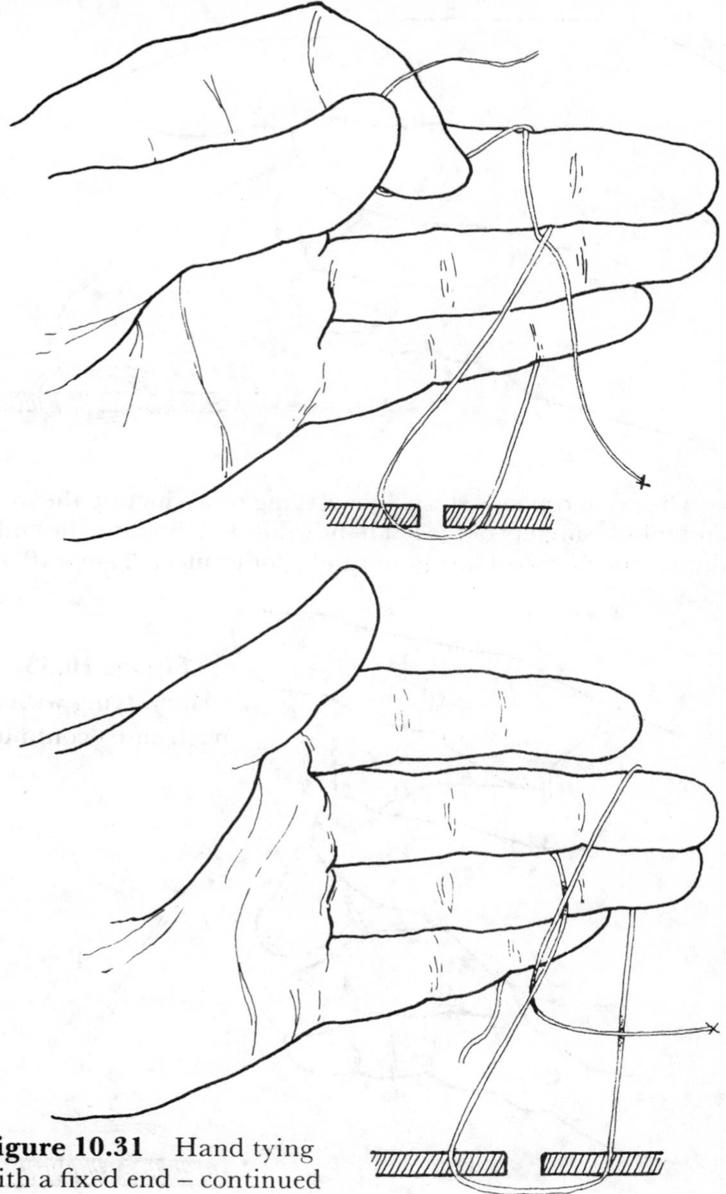

Figure 10.31 Hand tying with a fixed end – continued

Figure 10.32 Hand tying with a fixed end – continued

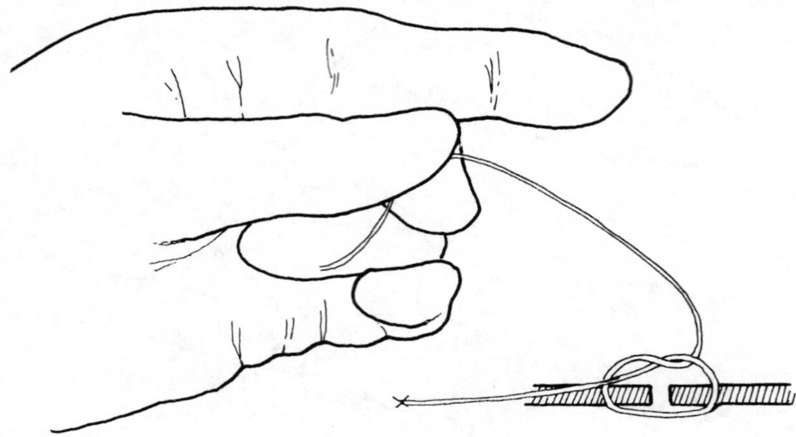

The second phase starts by splaying or abducting the index and middle fingers of the left hand while still holding the end of the free end between the thumb and middle finger (Figure 10.33).

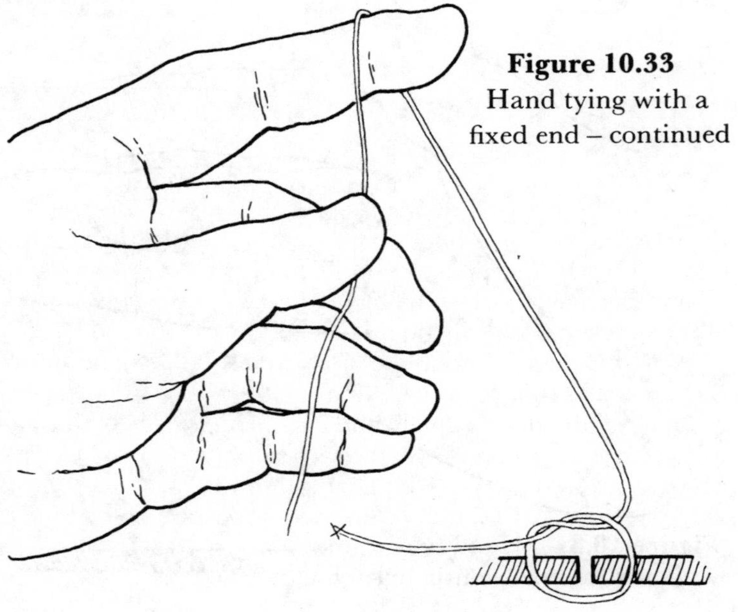

Figure 10.33 Hand tying with a fixed end – continued

The line is now lying across the gap between the index and middle finger. The fixed end is then brought up by the right hand to cross it from behind to in front (Figure 10.34).

Figure 10.34 Hand tying with a fixed end – continued

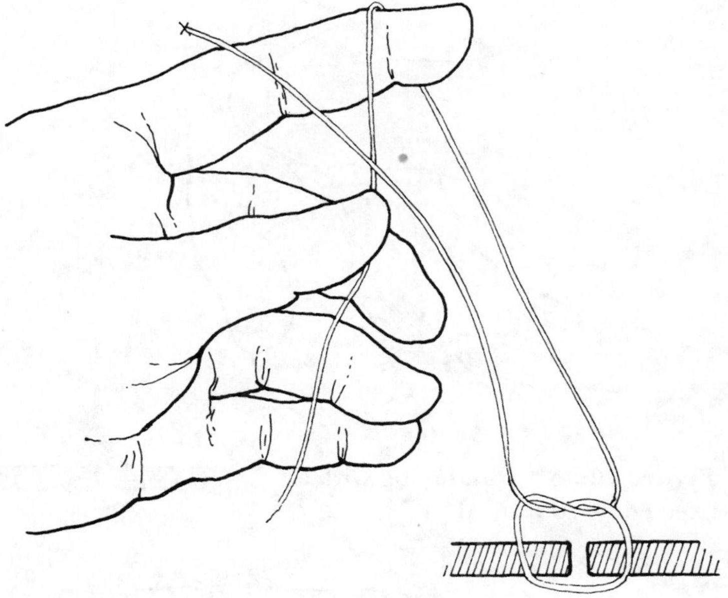

The index finger now hooks above the fixed line and under the free line and as it hooks back and to the left, the free line is released by the thumb and middle finger and is drawn through behind the fixed line now being held between the opposing sides of the index and middle finger. (See Figures 10.35 to 10.37.)

When through, this can be grasped normally again between the index and thumb and the final phase of the knot completed.

Once again, descriptively and even with the aid of diagrams, this seems a very complicated series of manoeuvres, but a piece of string around the thigh and a few minutes' practice following the diagrams, is all that is needed to start to get this as a perfectly natural series of movements about which one does not have to think consciously in each individual part.

Figure 10.35 Hand tying with a fixed end – continued

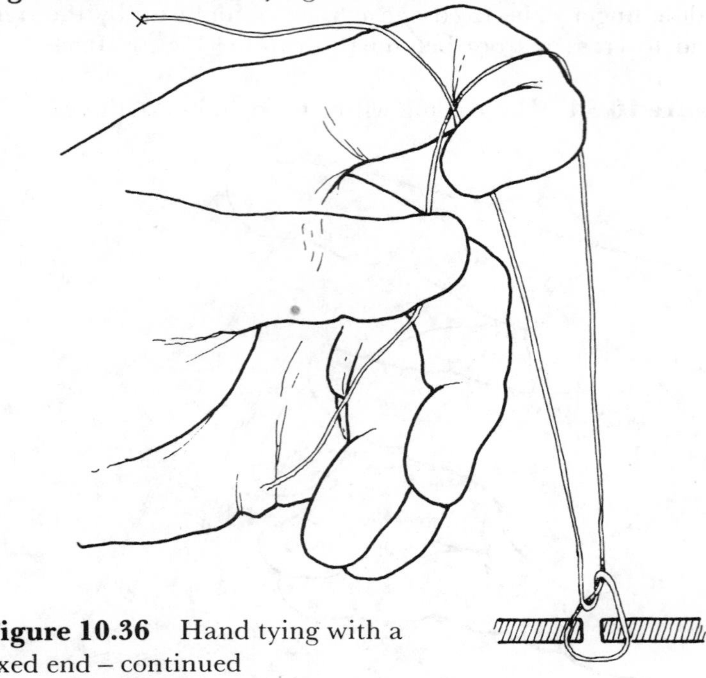

Figure 10.36 Hand tying with a fixed end – continued

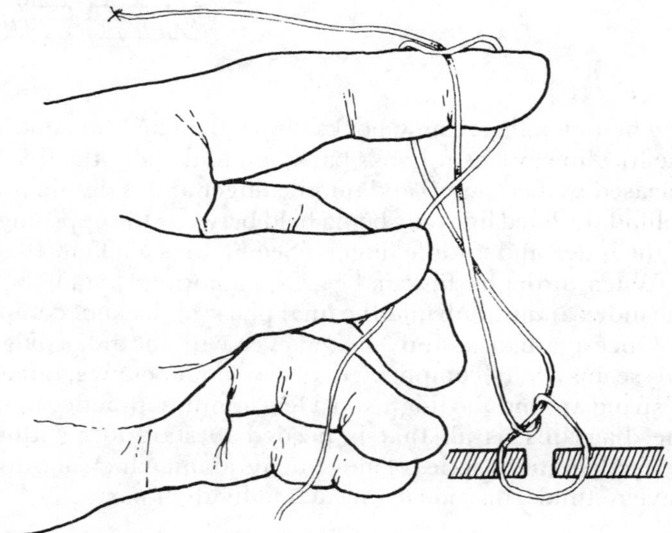

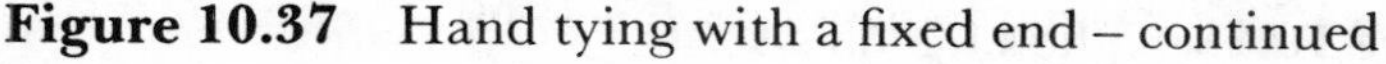

Figure 10.37 Hand tying with a fixed end – continued

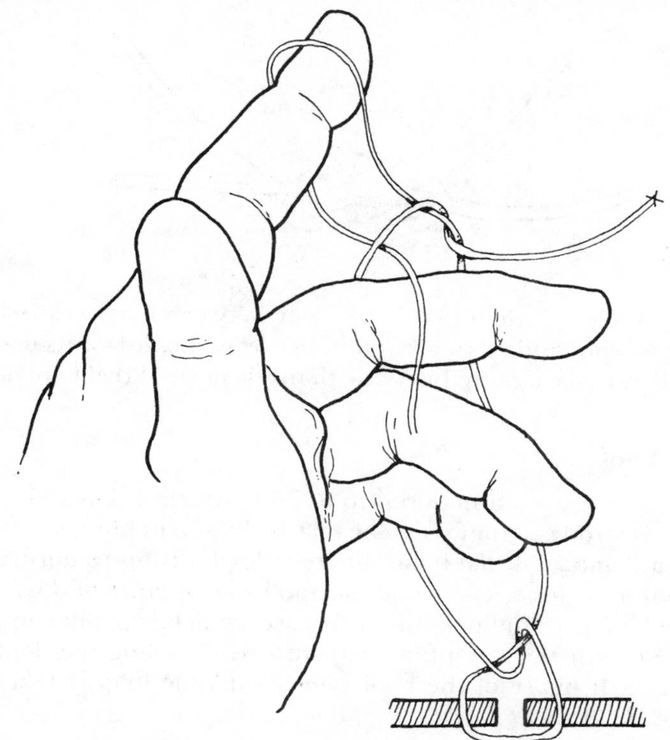

The surgeon's knot

This is a modification of the reef knot which is used by a great number of surgeons as it has the property of 'holding' a little firmer at the end of the first phase before the second phase of the reef knot is completed.

It is quite simple to do insomuch that instead of doing one loop around for the first phase of the reef knot there are two loops (Figure 10.38).

This double loop does mean that when the first stage of the stitch is tensioned, it does tend to hold that bit better before the normal second phase of the reef knot is added to it to lock it in place.

Figure 10.38 The surgeon's knot

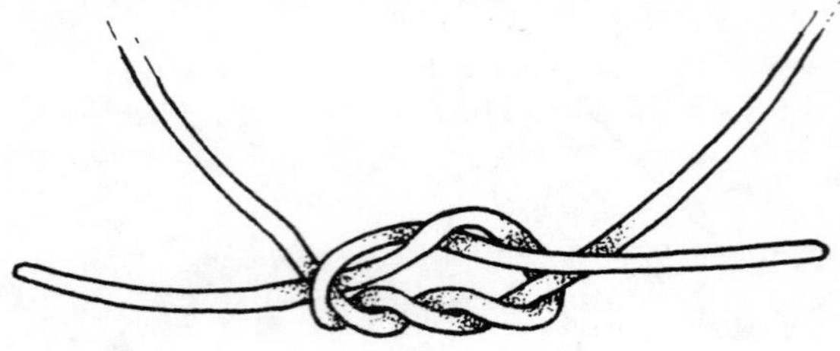

It is, in fact, a stitch that is half way between a nylon stitch and a reef knot and has a great number of advocates for its use, but it does make a more bulky tie than the normal reef knot.

Nylon knot

Nylon is a very good material to use for suturing skin as it is inert, it is strong so that it can be relatively thin in bore, but its one disadvantage is that it has inherent flexibility and a normal reef knot may just become undone and loose because of this.

This being so, the nylon knot is used, which is similar to a reef knot with the exception that instead of taking one loop around each phase of the knot tying, a double loop is taken (Figure 10.39).

Figure 10.39 Nylon knot

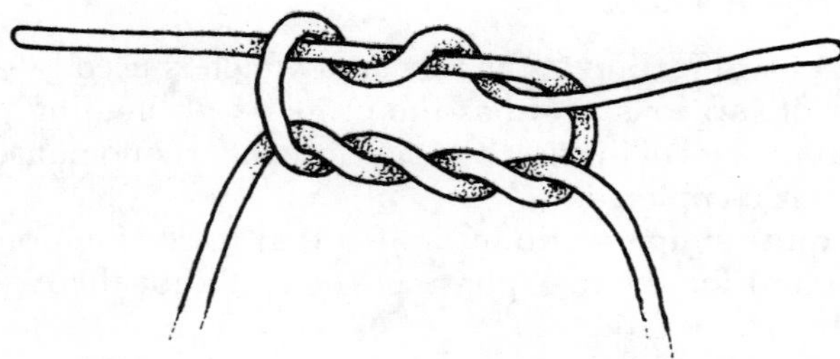

This resulting knot is a little more bulky than the reef knot, but it is a much more secure knot to tie for nylon and with that material should always be used.

Tightening the knot

Although it seems simplistic to be making the point about tying the knot a specific entity in this chapter, it is in fact very important that the basic principle of the two ends of the knot being tightened opposing each other is always remembered. This means that if the knot is on the skin level, the fingers can hold the ligature or suture and by lateral tension it will tighten, and one element is tightening it up against the other (Figure 10.40).

Figure 10.40 Correct tightening of the knot with the ends opposing each other

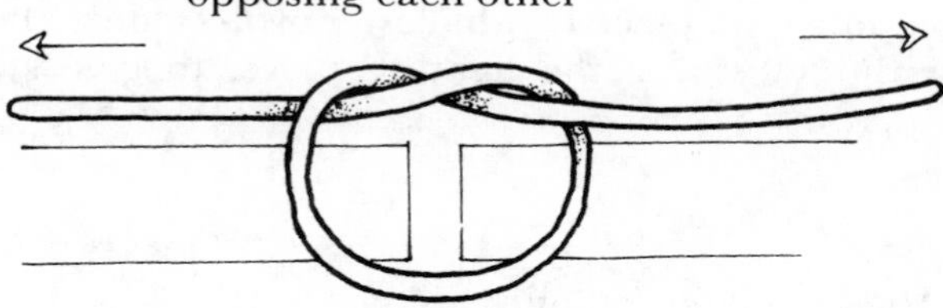

It is, however, very easy to try to tighten the knot by pulling as in Figure 10.41 where not only is the knot being tightened, but also the tissues through which the stitch or suture has been placed is also being subjected to abnormal tensioning which may result in it tearing through the tissues.

Figure 10.41 Incorrect tightening of the knot resulting in abnormal tensioning in the tissues

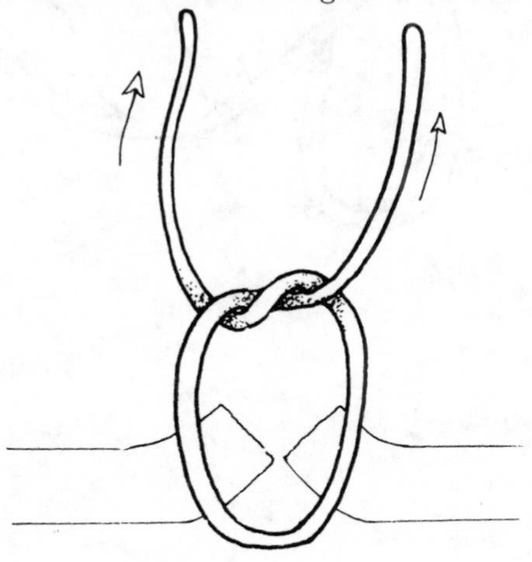

In those cases where it is impossible to get a horizontal pull on each side, one side must be held firmly with the finger or needle holder held right up against the knot, then the tensioning is done by pulling on the other side. This means that the finger holding the end near the knot is stopping any tenting of the tissues underneath and although the tensioning carried out on the other side is at an angle it is still being pulled directly against the finger and the suture material held in it.

It does not matter whether the knot is being tied with instruments or with the fingers, if in fact the horizontal tensioning cannot be achieved, then either the instrument or the finger must be placed right low down against the knot grasping the suture or the ligature there, to give stability (Figure 10.42).

Figure 10.42 Giving stability to the knot

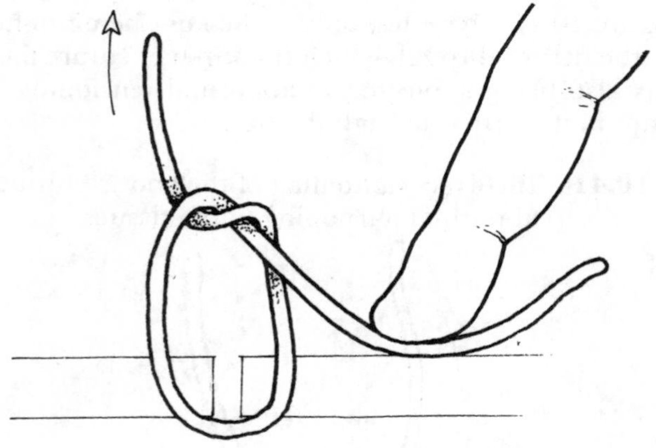

CHAPTER 11

Theatre Organisation and Procedure

Instruments

Having handled, considered and then selected instruments to use out of the variety that have been suggested, the assembling of these instruments into sets must now be organised.

A standard set is the grouping of the basic instruments that are going to be used for most procedures. The advantages of having a standard set are:

1. The same set can be put out and sterilised by an inexperienced person who does not need to know anything of the specifics of the operation to be performed.
2. Just as the standard set of instruments is the same that is put out each time, it is also the same that is checked in at the end of the operation each time so any discrepancy is very much more easily spotted.

   The likelihood of leaving an instrument in a patient with this type of surgery is remote. However, the likelihood of an unchecked instrument being discarded with soiled dressings and towels into an incinerator, is much higher.
3. The combination of each person's individual set will vary but, once established, its constituent parts should be either listed in the instrument cupboard, or a drawing, showing each individual instrument and how the set is to be, should be made and displayed.

   It may be advantageous, in fact, not only to have the list of the instruments but also to have the drawing in the instrument cupboard at the same time.
4. The storage of the instruments, as discussed earlier, should be in a constant place and, if possible, they should once again be stored as sets to minimise omissions and to make the checking procedure much easier.

> There is nothing more frustrating than reaching for an instrument half way through a procedure and finding it still resides in the instrument cupboard.

Having established the basic standard set, there may be extras needed for specific procedures. It is better to keep the standard set with as many things in it as are likely to be needed, and the specials and additions as limited as possible.

The specials will mainly relate to syringes, special needles, medicut, etc.

The more standard the technique the more adept and competent the surgeon becomes at refining it. A technique which varies on each occasion may lead to problems and a slipshod result.

Towel packs and drapes

The modern advent of prepacked towels, which are sterile, made of paper and disposable at the end of the operation, are a total boon for this type of surgery, especially when the facility for washing, packing and sterilising regular linen towels is nonexistent.

The prepacked towels come in various formats and in order to keep the variety and storage problems at a minimum there are two groups to be considered. There is the towelling of the trolley and the towelling of the patient.

The trolley

A towel pack is needed for the trolley. The pack must be packed and sterilised so that the sterile contents of the pack can be released from the unsterile packet and put on the trolley surface. Once the sterile pack is on the trolley it can be opened, either by the operator who is scrubbed up, gloved up and sterile, or by a sterile assistant who is fully scrubbed up before the operation.

The pack should open and the towel, when unfolded, should cover and overlap the trolley edges.

This sterile towel is the essential basis for setting-up on, but it can be refined in various ways.

(a) If the trolley drape is just a simple towel then, along with the instruments that are next transferred from the steriliser to the trolley, there must also be two sterile porringers and a sterile kidney dish, all being essential to put lotions in or to receive debris. There must also be a facility for adding sterile swabs from a similar prepacked pack on to the trolley.

Whichever system is preferred, these extra prepacked, sterile, separate swabs are always needed and should always be available. Therefore, with this system, a towel for the trolley is prepacked by itself. Some feel it is an advantage to have a sterile kidney dish in the steriliser with the porringers so that the instruments can be placed in the kidney dish and transferred in that way from the steriliser to the trolley.

(b) The trolley towel pack is prepared by some firms, and not only is there the towel, but also a sterile, disposable kidney dish and porringers, a few swabs and perhaps a small plastic tray. Quite often disposable forceps are included as well, which need not be used.

The advantage of these prepacked sets is that, at the end of the operation, it is all disposable. It is also very convenient to have everything present when the towels are unfolded. However, these packs are more expensive and it is still necessary to have the extra sterile swab packs available.

Summary of trolley towels

1. Prepacked sterile towel pack to cover and overlap the edges of the trolley and using a sterile kidney dish and porringers which are sterilised with the instruments and can be used to transfer the instruments from the steriliser to the trolley top.

   Or, alternatively, similar sterile towel pack with the addition of an enclosed, disposable kidney dish and porringers.
2. Sterile packets of swabs available, whichever system is used.

The choice must be a personal one, but the simple pack with the sterilised kidney dish and porringers being added from the steriliser has stood the test of time and is favoured, particularly as these simple towel trolley covers can be used in a different region, as will be seen later.

The Patient

Having assembled the trolley with its sterile surface, various dishes and instruments, and after cleaning the operative site, the area must also be towelled off.

There is a multiplicity of different sizes and combinations of prepacked, disposable, sterile towels on the market, and the options have to be refined down to the fewest varieties that are necessary and best for the job.

1. The simplest is a medium-sized towel with a precut hole which gives access to the operative site. This is very simple, very functional and can be used in a variety of operations as the hole can be enlarged if necessary to increase the range of its uses. These towels should be considered as the standard for most procedures.

   There is a variety of different firms offering various refinements, such as adhesive at the side, etc., and the specific design must be one of personal choice, but the concept of having a single towel with a hole in it appeals most and should be stocked.

2. However, there are procedures where more access is needed than can be provided by the single hole. Specifically when local tying and manipulating the leg, emptying distal veins before injection, or tying of varicose veins, where two ties at different and widespread sites may be necessary.

   These cases have to be towelled up by using a combination of rectangular towels both under and around the leg, etc. Once again there are multiple choices of specialist sets, but to store and finance these is neither practical nor feasible and it is best to use a constant drape for these cases. If the trolley drape is the single one with no added disposables, then the same packet and format of drape can be used as a patient drape in these bigger cases.

   This cuts down storage, cuts down variety, etc., and has a great deal to recommend it.

Summary of patient drapes

1. The majority are covered by a drape with a hole at its centre, the exact size, shape and design being a matter of choice.

2. Some procedures need more extensive draping and if the simple towel is being used for the trolley top, the same type of towel can be used as the drapes for the more extensive type of patient towelling.
   This eases the problems of ordering, problems of storage, etc., and should be considered.
3. If it is preferred to drape the trolley with towels containing disposable pots, then a separate supply of simple, rectangular, prepacked sterile towels must also be kept for the extensive patient drapes.
4. There are special drape packs for cases such as catheterisation etc., but it is not recommended that these be stored and used as the draping system described, although simple they are perfectly adequate to cover these eventualities.

Pre-operative preparation

The sterilisation of instruments in a set with the possible sterilisation of kidney dish and sponges has now been discussed.

The trolley top has been draped by emptying the prepacked sterile towel on to it. It has been opened and arranged by the scrubbed up assistant, and the standard instrument setting (see p. 48), once sterilised, has been transferred to the trolley and laid out as specified in the diagram by the surgeon. Extra swabs have been emptied on to the trolley.

At this point it is necessary to add:

(a) needles
(b) sutures
(c) blades
(d) syringes
(e) injecting needles

It is here that the surgeon's personal preference must be known and stipulated. It is of little use advising more than in general terms, as has been done, what should be available.

The best scheme is to start a small card index, that can be kept in the instrument cupboard, for the additional needles, etc., which are needed for any specific operations.

This index will be altered and amended as experience and time goes on. If it is there the person setting up the trolley for any specific operation can refer to it and then empty on to the trolley sterile needles, etc., stipulated on the list as being needed. This saves time and also gives a much more professional appearance to the whole surgical procedure.

Timing

If the trolley if fully laid up and the procedure is not due to start for a while, the top of the trolley must be covered by a sterile towel until both the patient and the surgeon are in the theatre.

This avoids contamination with dust or by being brushed against by any passing person.

CHAPTER 12

Specific Operations

Skin lesions
- Pigmented moles
- Rodent ulcers or basal cell carcinoma
- Seborrheic warts
- Sebaceous cyst

Varicose veins

Venous flares

Toe-nail surgery
- Removal of toe-nail
- Acute subungual haematoma
- Ablation of toe-nail bed
- Lateral nail-bed ablation

Local excisions
- Local excision of a lipoma
- Lymph gland biopsy
- Mucous cyst of mouth or ranula

Ganglia

Surgery of bursae
- Olecranon bursa
- Infra-patella bursa
- Pre-patella bursa

Trauma

Vasectomy

Aspiration of cyst of breast

Drainage of a hydrocele

Catheterisation

Thrombosed external pile or peri-anal haematoma

Skin lesions

Pigmented moles

This is a generic description used for pigmented skin lesions which can be divided histologically and clinically into two groups:

1. Pigmented naevi
2. Malignant melanoma

All pigmented lesions of the skin fill every doctor with apprehension and these lesions are very common in all age groups.

The vast majority are benign, yet the remaining small percentage are either premalignant or, in the case of the malignant melanoma, outrageously virulently malignant from the outset. Despite all the advances made in the science of oncology over recent years the specific attack on this tumour cytotoxically still has a great way to progress.

The problem therefore arises as to the diagnosis in the first instance. The initial definitive line of attack is essentially a surgical policy.

The treatment of malignant melanoma which are clinically malignant from the outset or are highly suspicious of being so, is surgical and that treatment involves wide removal by a margin of at least 3 cm from the edge of the tumour, or from the site of the most peripheral satellite.

Following the removal the area is grafted.

The old maxim that a malignant melanoma has not been properly removed if there is a resultant scar and not a graft, is 99 per cent accurate since wide undercutting and mobilisation of skin following a wide excision of a melanoma is bad surgical practice as it opens up wide tissue planes to potential problems.

It therefore follows that any pigmented lesion that is clinically thought to be malignant should be referred urgently to a consultant surgeon who can treat it radically under general anaesthetic and investigate it fully at the outset.

The criteria for this referral must be based on the following clinical points and following exclusion of these cases, a wide variety of pigmented lesions remain. A number of these need excision properly to re-assure both the doctor and the patient and particularly because some will be falling into the histological bracket of a junctional naevus. This is a possible premalignant condition for subsequest development of a malignant melanoma.

Indications for referral due to probability to malignancy are:

1. Size – patients are surprisingly perceptive about increasing size in a lesion which they can see, but it must be remembered that the common site of occurrence of a malignant melanoma is either on the back or the sole of the foot. These are both difficult places for the patient to assess.
2. Character change of the lesion itself:
   - (a) Bleeding can be due to trauma but even if the lesion looks totally benign and there is even a small history of trauma it should not be given any benefit of the doubt but should be excised.
   - (b) Nodularity – an irregularity which may eventually lead to ulceration.
   - (c) Ulceration of a previously flat lesion.
   - (d) Irritation – itching or irritation means mandatory immediate surgery.
   - (e) Change of colour – a history of getting darker or more pigmented which, when it occurs, is often noted by the patient.
   - (f) A change of character of the surrounding skin. If satellite nodules or pigmented areas occur in the skin around the lesion this is highly suspicious of malignancy.
   - (g) Special site – any subungual pigmented lesion should be deemed to be malignant.

All of these clinical characteristics make it mandatory to refer the patient.

The remaining group of pigmented naevi do sometimes need excision, even though clinically not malignant and falling into the above criteria.

Any pigmented lesion which, for any reason, causes it to be brought to the attention of the doctor, even apologetically as being 'making a fuss about nothing', should be excised.

Any lesion that is subjected to recurrent trauma or any lesion that is pigmented and on the back or sole of the foot and which has occasioned a visit to the doctor for an opinion is virtually self diagnostic. It should be removed and subjected to histological examination.

Importance should also be attached to any pigmented lesion where the colour varies in different areas of the surface.

The vast majority of these will inevitably turn out to be benign intradermal naevi. Very occasionally a junctional naevus may be removed which is potentially malignant.

Juvenile melanoma

Melanoma prepubertally very rarely turn malignant so, in contradistinction to those in the puberty and older age groups, can be treated a little more conservatively. However, if any is causing anxiety at all, it is best referred to a dermatological consultant for his opinion and advice. Certainly this is preferable to trying to excise or remove these in Outpatients under local anaesthetic.

Anaesthetic

If there is a liability of distortion of the skin local infiltration around the lesion may necessitate drawing the proposed lines of incision on the skin. This should be done with a skin pencil before infiltration.

Surgical instruments

A general set.

Surgical technique

Any skin lesion has to be excised with an elliptical incision taking an area of skin outside the lesion on each side. The area of normal skin need be only 2 to 3 mm but the edge of the lesion must be totally cleared.

Siting of the direction of the ellipse is of paramount importance unless, for some technical reason, the ellipse is being directly dictated by the lesion.

To obtain a good scar at the end of the excision, mentally draw a line through the lesion in the site of election which a single incision would take, ie in one of Langer's lines where the maximal tension is end to end and the minimum tension is side to side.

After noting the direction of that line of election, the ellipse is then removed with the point of the ellipse at each end being situated on that line.

If the point at each end of the ellipse is situated on that line and if the distance from the centre of the ellipse to the line is the same on each side, then when the ellipse of skin is removed the edges should be both equidistant in length and subsequently lie in the line of least tension, giving the best scar.

Most of the surgical technique has already been described under general surgical technique. However the points to be remembered are that the skin must be incised at right angles to the skin. The incision should go deeply, totally through the skin and should take some of the underlying fatty tissue with it so that an elliptical block of tissue is removed.

Following the removal and haemostasis being established the deep fat can be approximated with 40 atraumatic catgut on a half-circle needle and skin stitches with inter-digitating steristrip straps being applied for skin closure.

The block of tissue fat and ellipse of skin containing the lesion is sent off for histological examination *in toto*.

★ ★ ★

Rodent ulcers or basal cell carcinoma

The alternative forms of treatment for a rodent ulcer are radiotherapy or surgery.

The clinical features of the ulcer are of its origins as a small pearly type of nodule. Later, when it become larger, it ulcerates and has a raised, rolled edge.

The majority of rodent ulcers occur on exposed surfaces — the upper part of the face, the scalp, the hands and sometimes the arms. It is for this reason that only a few are suitable for surgery under local anaesthetic in this particular operative context. This is because surgery of facial lesions, where the scar is of paramount importance, does sometimes require more definitive skills or a general anaesthetic.

However, rodent ulcers may present on the back of the hand or on the scalp, either of which are amenable to surgery under local anaesthetic. Their treatment in those situations will be exactly the same as described later for pigmented naevi, but, overall, the majority of these lesions will be referred on, either for definitive surgery or for radiotherapy.

★ ★ ★

Seborrheic warts

Seborrheic warts are common, benign, sessile lesions which, in the middle aged and elderly age groups, cause cosmetic embarrassment. Sometimes, due to their susceptibility to trauma, they also become painful and bleed.

Due to their wide base, treatment with excision does mean relatively extensive surgery. Due to this and their usual multiplicity, treatment by freezing with carbon dioxide snow is uncomfortable and not totally successful.

However, surgical treatment which involves removing the wart and the superficial layer of the epidermis is quite successful, particularly for the more extensive lesions which are more difficult to destroy with freezing.

The additional advantage of removing the lesion surgically is that it does enable the surgeon to obtain a definitive histological examination and confirmation of the diagnosis following the surgery.

Position on the table

This is dependent on the site.

Instruments

A small blade, preferably a rounded shape
Swabs
Haemostatic sponge such as Sterispon or Surgicel should be available

Anaesthesia

Local infiltration under the lesion.

Operative technique

After establishing anaesthesia, preparing the skin and towelling, a small bladed 15 type of shaped blade is slowly swept across the surface of the skin.

The knife blade is held only slightly off the vertical with the handle parallel to the skin. This means that the pressure and force applied is more across and parallel to the skin surface rather than down and cutting into it.

The object is more to scrape the lesion off the surface of the skin rather than to cut into the skin and excise it. The sweeping action should start peripherally and move into the centre and then a new stroke made further round the periphery with the same direction of movement. It is repeated in the same way, rather like going round the outside of a clock face and moving into the centre.

The result of this is to remove the seborrheic wart and leave a raw surface with multiple tiny bleeding points on it.

This is the same appearance as that which follows taking a thin Thiersch graft.

Haemostasis is secured in the first instance with pressure via a swab and, if after due time, this is not successful, pressure on top of a haemostatic sponge dressing such as Surgicel or Sterispon, may be needed.

The haemostatic sponge is left in place with its attendant clot.

A non-adhesive dressing is applied on top of the Surgicel and, if possible, pressure is applied on top of that.

The result as far as recurrence is concerned is usually very good and the resulting area may be a little paler than the surrounding skin cosmetically. However, this is preferable to a long scar or a similar cosmetic change that would have resulted if the wart had been excised or burnt off with CO_2 snow.

Post-operatively

The dressing and Sterispon should be left in place for 48 hours. The non-adhesive overlying dressing is then removed. If the underlying Sterispon or haemostatic sponge is dry, it is left. Otherwise it is soaked off and a new non-adhesive, non-occlusive dressing applied.

Pathology

All warts of whatever clinical diagnosis must be subjected to histological examination. This is one of the advantages of removing the lesion rather than destroying the tissue with freezing.

If more than one wart is removed each must be sent separately and accurately labelled for histological examination. This is so that in the eventuality of one being suspect, its exact site of origin is known rather than it being one wart out of several in the same container.

⋆ ⋆ ⋆

Sebaceous cyst

Probably the most common lump that a surgeon is asked to diagnose is the sebaceous cyst. It seems to be a fact of life that patients tend to put up with one or more multiple sebaceous cysts for a long time before seeking diagnosis and treatment. They do not seem to equate its appearance with the possibility of a malignancy, perhaps because someone else in the family has had one before and has reassured them.

Usually occurring on the scalp or ear, they present in an assortment of sizes and multiplicity. A well-developed cyst is easier to remove than a very small one which gets 'lost', or a large one where bleeding and the extent of the infiltration needed sometimes presents problems.

Indications for removal are related to recurrent infection or cosmetic.

1. Infected sebaceous cyst

If infection occurs in the cyst it appears to be a very good culture medium; an abscess forms rapidly with surrounding cellulitis.

If the skin of the abscess has not burst through the punctum to allow it to discharge, it may have to be incised in order to allow the discharge of sebaceous material and pus.

As there is usually an associated cellulitis, a course of antibiotics should be given.

No attempt should be made to treat the sebaceous cyst definitively at this stage as any attempt to curette the cavity or other dramatics will stand a good chance of spreading infection and not have the desired ultimate effect.

The infection should be controlled, settled and only when totally quiescent should it be reassessed for definitive excision.

2. **Uninfected sebaceous cyst**

Indications for surgery are usually cosmetic, or a past history of infection. If there is any doubt in patients' minds they should be immediately reassured that it is neither malignant nor a pre-malignant condition.

Shaving

In the past, wide areas of the scalp used to be shaved around the cyst, but this practice has been shown to be unnecessary from the infective point of view, although it does make it more difficult from the technical view point if shaving does not take place.

Surgical anatomy

The sebaceous glands are situated in the corium, and the ducts open usually in a hair follicle and the secretion is mainly sebum.

A cystic swelling was thought to be due to a blockage of the duct with resultant build-up of the sebaceous material behind it. The resultant wax-containing cystic swelling always has a punctum on the skin which is not necessarily obviously associated with a hair follicle.

Instruments

General set.

Position on the table

Varied, but must be comfortable for the patient and provide access for the surgeon. It is sometimes necessary to have the head over a pillow or on one side or the other, or, alternatively, it may be necessary to put the pillow in the nape of the neck to support the head being flexed in order to get at a cyst near the occiput.

Anaesthesia

Infiltration around the cyst with 1% Lignocaine and Adrenalin. The Adrenalin tends to constrict the small vessels of the scalp which are very numerous and cut down any bleeding.

Surgical technique

1. With a small cyst ensure the punctum is marked with an indelible skin pencil before infiltrating, as the infiltration itself, around the scalp, makes it impossible to feel the cyst afterwards and it can very easily get 'lost'.
2. Before sterilising the skin, or injecting the local anaesthetic, get an ordinary bar of soap, wet it and then use this to smear down the hair around the cyst so that it is lying radially away from the cyst and is held by the soft soap. This helps to stop the hair getting involved in the operation and is well worthwhile taking care about before starting the procedure.

   Another way to control the hair is by using broad Elastoplast, but this usually sticks only to the hairs on the outside and those underneath very soon intrude on the operative field. The soap method is usually considered the best.

   Following cleansing of the skin, an injection of the local anaesthetic is administered.

The incision

The incision is transverse from one side to the other across the centre of the cyst, and is always elliptical in shape enclosing the punctum.

The size of the ellipse depends how globular and how protruberant the cyst is. The width of the ellipse which is excised with the punctum and with the cyst, should be a size that means the remaining edges when the cyst is removed, lie without tension and without having any redundant skin.

It is very tempting to think that a thin ellipse should be taken and that the skin can always be trimmed up afterwards if it is redundant, but although this seems to be easy it does, in fact, present more problems, and is not as easy to get right at the end as it is if one estimates it fully to start with.

Estimation of the width of the ellipse

If the cyst seems to be protruberant from the surface of the scalp by half its diameter, then the ellipse from side to side, centred on the punctum, should on each side be about one-third of the distance from the punctum to the perimeter, thus leaving two-thirds of the distance from the edge of the ellipse on each side to the perimeter. See Figure 12.1.

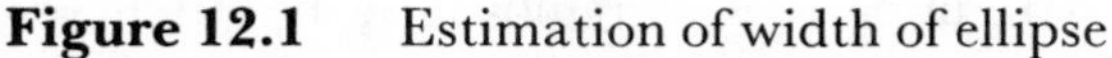

Figure 12.1 Estimation of width of ellipse

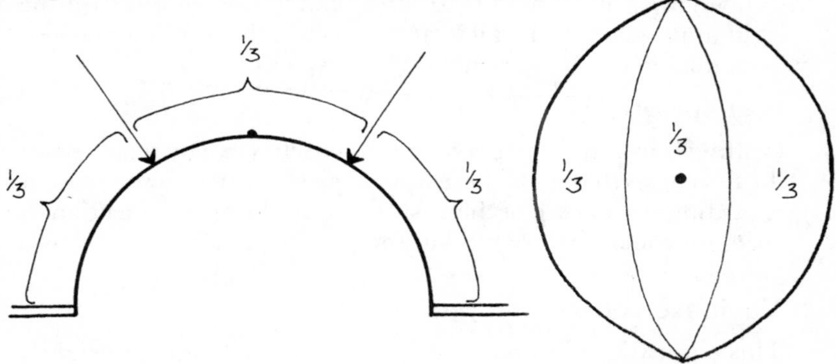

The incision of the ellipse is gently cut until the white of the cyst capsule is seen in its depth.

The outer side of the skin can be retracted with a fine skin hook, and the skin ellipse around the punctum can be held with Russian Mayo-type forceps. The plane around the capsule is developed with opening and closing artery forceps until, with gentle pressure on each side, the cyst will present itself apart from a little deep adventitia through the incision.

No attempt should be made to grasp the actual capsule of the cyst itself, as inevitably this results in its rupture which distorts the whole operation.

The deep adventitia can usually be either divided or clipped depending on whether it has many vessels in it. If it is clipped it should then be tied with 40 plain catgut.

The skin flaps, which remain from the skin overlying the cyst, are now closed with through-and-through stitches. If there is any oozing then mattress stitches may have to be used to control it a little better.

As a pressure dressing in the hair is virtually impossible, the operative field must be dry before closing.

Whichever type of stitch is used, there are two important factors to remember.

1. Leave the ends of the stitches long after tying. This will help the surgeon to find them when they are being removed.
2. Note how many stitches are put in.

Both these points are important as removal of the stitches is difficult with matted hair around, and it does not create the right impression if a recalcitrant stitch which has remained and been missed has to be removed some weeks later.

Post-operatively

Healing is usually very good and the stitches can be removed on the fifth to sixth day. If there is any apprehension in the patient regarding the nature of the cyst, it should be sent for section in order for the necessary reassurance.

* * *

Varicose veins

This clinical condition is one of tortuouis, distended, unsightly veins of the legs causing cosmetic symptoms and associated with aching and oedema of the ankle and the leg. There is also the increased risk of damage to the vein due to trauma, and the increased risk of phlebitis developing.

The distension in the veins is due to back pressure of the column of venous blood in a segment of vein which has lost is valves.

When the peripheral muscular pump compresses the vein and propels the blood centrally, it is not supported then by any valves when the pump relaxes and the blood comes back. This back pressure causes the symptoms and puts further stress on any remaining competent valves below the column.

The treatment is directed at isolating the normal system from the abnormal.

If the long saphenous system from its junction with the femoral vein in the inguinal region has lost its valves and the whole system is abnormal, then there is no way that either local ties or injections are going to do any good and, in fact, may do harm.

The isolation of the long saphenous with the normal deep femoral vein has got to be carried out flush at their junction. All the local branches of the femoral vein which may well subsequently distend and bypass this junction, have to be divided.

This cannot be done by injection as the danger of getting sclerosant in a deep vein is catastrophic; this cannot be done by local tie of the long saphenous somewhere near the junction as experience has confirmed that this will always recur.

Therefore, the only treatment for long saphenous or short saphenous system incompetence is definitive, well-performed surgery under general anaesthetic in hospital, which gives most satisfying results to patients and surgeons alike.

Coming one layer peripherally, however, in the vascular tree where the underlying long saphenous system is normal with intact valves (but one or more branches or segments coming off this long saphenous have lost their valves and become varicose) the surgeon is then in a situation where local isolation of the varicose segment branching from the normal underlying long saphenous or short saphenous vein can be carried out.

Once that site is controlled all the peripheral, distended tortuous vein then has the back pressure removed from it. It can then be obliterated and the symptoms dramatically improved.

Having treated this abnormal branch, if the underlying long saphenous or short saphenous is itself normal then there is no reason at all why this should recur.

This is a very satisfactory procedure for the surgeon and the patient, but it does depend on a diagnosis being accurately made, that the underlying long saphenous system is normal and it is only the branches coming off it that are abnormal with pathological valves.

The same procedure as described in pre-operative marking should be carried out in the original examination of the leg in order to isolate clinically the pathological section and to be able to make an accurate diagnosis.

In summary, injection and local ties of varicosities, or a combination of both, is reserved for those patients who have a clinically sound underlying long or short saphenous system and have a group of abnormal varicosities draining from one segment of that system.

If those varicosities are isolated and treated by whichever method, the underlying system is left intact and a good result should be obtained.

The size of the varicosities, governs whether the treatment should be:

1. Sclerosant injection with compression alone, or
2. A local tie of the vein to isolate the pathological section associated with sclerosant injection in the collapsed vein distal to this and compression of that vein.

Long saphenous system

The branches of the long saphenous system usually affected are:

1. *Medial or anterior vein of the lower leg*
   This drains up from the lateral side of the ankle and then crosses medially as it ascends and joins the long saphenous just above the knee-joint line on the medial side of the knee.
2. *Parasaphenous vein*
   This runs in the medial side of the thigh with its upper limit in the mid-thigh region.
   It runs down alongside the long saphenous and has branches in the lower below-knee region and is cosmetically very disfiguring.
   It is usually fed from an incompetent mid-thigh perforating vein going directly through to the femoral system deeply although, on occasions, a similar distended varicosity does arise in this region originating from the long saphenous itself.
3. *The lateral vein of the leg*
   This drains from the lateral side of the lower leg, up the lateral side of the knee and across the front of the thigh into the anterior thigh vein complex which then joins the long saphenous at a variable distance below the sapheno-femoral opening, although it might drain directly into the femoral vein itself.
4. *The medial thigh vein*
   Draining from the posterior part of the thigh round the medial side of the thigh to join the long saphenous usually about 10 cms below the sapheno-femoral junction.

Short saphenous system

The branches of the short saphenous system are usually unnamed and, with one exception, are not quite so constant.

This exception is a vein that joins with the short saphenous in the mid-calf region where it perforates the deep fascia and leads to varicosities spreading over the posterior part of the calf and also going down the lateral side of the ankle.

Pre-operative marking

This should be carried out on the day before operation because of shaving, and then gone over just before surgery if the marks have become indistinct.

Marking is vitally important and must be done by the surgeon himself with a skin-marking pencil whose lines are not going to be removed by the spirit in the skin paintup. Amongst commercial markers is Perm Marker by Venus or Tempo or an ordinary Pentel rolling writer pen which has a spirit-resistant ink.

It is not a good practice to use a skin-marking pencil which puts a layer of plastic on the skin as technically when the skin is being marked it is unsterile. Therefore, if the surgeon puts a plastic mark on the skin, then sterilises the skin around and over it, later cutting through that mark the knife-blade is, in fact, going through unsterilised skin.

The veins must be marked with the patient standing. The highest obvious part of the particular group of varicosities is found, and a small preliminary mark is made on the skin.

The patient then lies down, the leg is elevated and the blood massaged out of the limb. Then, with the limb still elevated, the preliminary mark is found and pressure applied with the thumb.

The patient then stands up with this pressure still being kept on. The vein below this feeder should remain empty, as retrograde filling has been stopped.

The aim and object is to find the highest, i.e. most central, point on the varicosity which is controlled by local pressure.

If no veins appear to fill higher up, then the mark is confirmed by drawing a line with the marking pen along each side of the vein with a transverse mark at the point where it is proposed that the incision should be made. (See Figure 12.2.)

Figure 12.2 Pre-operative marking

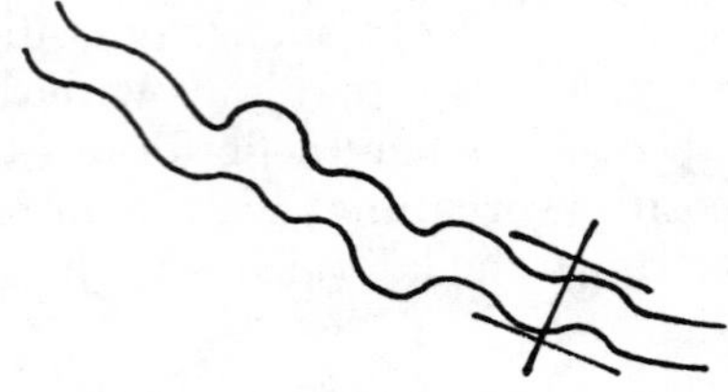

Having marked the top of the vein from its drainage source, it is often wise to make further marks of a similar type down the whole complex being treated. This is so that the surgeon can carry out a further local tie lower down with a further injection if necessary.

Remember that with the patient flat on the operating table, the distension of the vein disappears and the marks are the only lead one has. Therefore, they must be placed accurately and it saves time in the end if time is spent at the beginning by careful marking.

The number of ties and injections varies.

The total acceptable amount of injections to be used is one limiting factor as are the number of incisions that can be done under local anaesthetic in one session and, quite often, depending on the severity of the veins, more than one session may be needed.

Shaving

Shaving should cover 10 cms around each site and a 10 cm strip over the vein which joins the proposed site of upper and lower tie, if two are to be made, and below that site over the vein to be compressed.

Instruments

General set
+ 5 ccs syringe for sclerosant
+ Medicut needle or medium steel Injection hypodermic needle

Sutures
20 plain catgut ties
40 Mersilk on a cutting needle for skin

Blades
15 Gillette small handle only

Local anaesthetic

2% plain Lignocaine

Dressings

Sorbo-rubber triangular compression pad
Crepe bandages
Appropriate length of Tubigrip elastic tubular bandages or a fitted TED stocking

Lighting and position on table

The patient should be in a comfortable position which affords full access to the operative site.

The lights should be adjusted to cover the definite site of the first incision and also the possible site of any subsequent incision.

Operative technique

The area around the marks between the first mark and the second one to be operated upon is cleansed with skin preparation. The area peripherally below the lowest mark must also be cleansed so that the surgeon has access to the vein in its whole length the entire time. Having cleansed the the skin this area is then towelled off with four universal trolley towels.

As the quantities of local anaesthetic to be used are small, it is best to use 2% Plain Lignocaine without Adrenalin, and this is then drawn up into the 10 cc syringe. The subcutaneous area around the vein marks, to an area of about 3 cms in diameter, is infiltrated, taking great care not to harpoon the vein whilst so doing.

If a second incision is to be made lower down, this area is infiltrated at the same time.

It is worthwhile stressing at this point, once again, that all the local anaesthetic should be kept in a 10 cc syringe despite the amount to be used, and any sclerosant or toxic substance should always be in a 5 cc syringe to cut down the possibility of any confusion of the contents of any clear fluid in any syringe.

Skin incision

The surgeon always has the choice of the line of election to get an incision with the least tension across it, thereby giving a good scar — see Figure 12.3.

Figure 12.3 Skin incision to result in a good scar

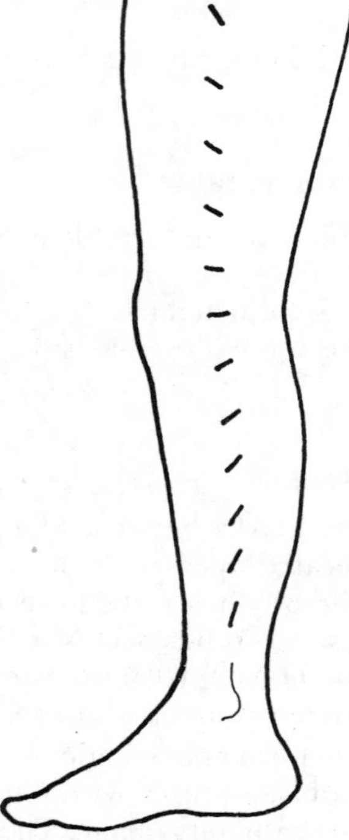

The maximum length of the incision should be 1 cm and preferably less.

Having gone through the skin over the vein, the vein is grasped firmly with a blunt-nosed artery forcep so that it does not tear. As it is lifted out of the incision slowly with the left hand, the right hand — using a pair of non-tooth dissecting forceps — clears any adherent fat off it so that it is completely clean.

An artery forcep is then introduced under it and opened. When this is through, the vein is bridged over the haemostat and is clear and clean.

The vein is then cleaned of fat both up and down as far as is practical under the skin edges in a similar way, taking great care not to injure it.

Having done this, a 30 plain catgut tie is drawn under the vein and tied as high as possible. This is facilitated by gentle downward traction on the vein as the tie is being secured.

The tie, having been knotted, is left about 5 cm long and an artery forcep is put on the two ends of catgut at that level as this provides a very useful and convenient hold, the excess catgut being cut off and retained.

A further 20 catgut tie is put under the vein and held but not tied at this stage.

The top incision is now complete and the vein is ready for injection.

The backflow of blood has been arrested so the vein below this can be emptied by rolling a swab along the vein with pressure down the leg as far as is feasible. Having emptied the vein, the assistant keeps pressure on it at that lower point.

This empty vein is now injected with sclerosant, which has previously been drawn up into the 5 cc syringe and has had the soft cannular part of the Medicut needle left in place, or, alternatively, has a small needle fitted.

The two holds of the vein are held with the left hand, as shown, which controls the vein and enables a small transverse cut to be made across the vein with fine scissors to the intima and the cannular, or a needle is threaded into the lumen.

The cannular element of a Medicut needle is preferred as it is soft and the risk of it going through the wall and out of the vein, resulting in sclerosant being injected subcutaneously, is reduced.

Once the cannular is in place, the lower catgut tie is secured around it and the vein to hold it there.

The vein can now be inspected and, if necessary, re-rolled to empty it of any blood that has seeped into it. Pressure is applied by an assistant at its lower end or the vein is tied at that point, empty, in a similar way. (See later.) Being empty, the sclerosant is injected, making sure that there is no extraversation locally.

This sclerosant is gently wiped along the vein down to the lower pressure point which is always maintained.

A further 30 plain catgut tie is now put under the vein and the cannular is removed. As it is pulled out, the vein is clipped with an artery forcep across the point where it was opened and the catgut tie just introduced is secured below that point.

The vein is then cut under the artery forcep, and the catgut tie on each cut end of the vein is cut short, at which point the ends of the vein usually retract into the incision.

The incision is closed with one or two mattress sutures of 40 Mersilk with Steristrip as additional support.

The sclerosant has now had several minutes in the long segment of empty vein.

A little Nobecutaine Spray is then applied on the incision and also on the skin along the course of the vein to the lower compression point. The vein is then covered with the triangular sorbo-rubber dressing over its full length down to the pressure point which is still maintained.

The Nobecutaine Spray on the skin tends to hold the sorbo-pad in place. The spray should never be used with any plastic padding, which tends to dissolve — it should be used only with the rubber.

A fine crepe bandage compressing the sorbo and the underlying vein can then be applied. Only when this is on and in place is the lower pressure point released.

More extensive veins

Sometimes with extensive varicosities it may be necessary to do a further tie at the lower pressure point, which will then allow a further long segment to be collapsed and injected.

Alternatively, any lower veins may be injected once the back pressure head has been removed with the local tie.

If two ties are planned at a long distance along the same complex, the procedure is modified.

Initially, both the sites are infiltrated with local anaesthetic. Having then exposed the vein in the upper more central incision as before and having got the cannular in place, the surgeon then moves to the lower site and repeats the process and mobilises the vein.

At this point the vein is under-run by a catgut tie but, as with the upper incision, this is not secured at this point.

The long segment of vein between the incisions is now emptied as before by rolling a swab over it. When it is empty the vein in the lower incision is bridged over forceps, keeping the whole long segment of vein between the two empty, and this is injected, as before. With the injection spread along its segment the upper incision is then closed.

The lower vein is then opened by a transverse cut and any excessive sclerosant can be milked out of the segment above it before the upper catgut tie on this vein, at this site, is secured.

The ends of this tie are once again left long, as before, to use as a hold.

The cannular is then once again put in the incision and fed down and tied with a catgut suture, as before.

The vein below this site is then emptied as far as is practicable and the procedure carried on as originally described, with the lower pressure point being maintained until the pressure bandage is applied over its full length.

Bandaging

When the skin incision is closed, the surgeon at that point, has the situation of a vein that has been emptied between the skin incision and tie, and the continuing pressure being applied lower down the vein. This whole segment of vein has been injected with sclerosant, and should have no blood in it.

That length of vein plus the upper skin incision is now sprayed with Nobecutaine Spray and the triangular sorbo-rubber pad is placed along the whole length of the vein from a point about 2.5 cm below the upper tie right down to the pressure on the vein distally that is still being maintained. Or, if a further tie has been done lower down, then the pad right down to approximately 2 cms proximal to that tie.

Having put the sorbo pad in place over the vein it is then held there by the adhesiveness of the Nobecutaine Spray.

At this point a tight, firm, crepe bandage is applied with sufficient tension around the pad and leg so that the pad itself is compressed down to the flat transverse contour. When this crepe is applied and secured with plaster, a rolled, appropriate size and length of Tubigrip elasticated stocking or a TED stocking is placed on top. The stocking should extend from the forefoot up to the upper part of the crepe bandage.

By compressing the vein this way it means that when the stitches are removed the compression bandage need not be disturbed even if two local ties have been carried out.

Post-operatively

Mobility is encouraged and the mechanism of the peripheral muscular pump is explained to the patient.

When the patient is vertical he should fidget and keep the leg muscles contracting and relaxing all the time and should not stand still and relax for any length of time without so doing.

Alternatively, when the patient is sitting the leg should be elevated on a stool to combat gravity. The leg should not hang over the edge of a chair, car seat or plane seat with gravity encouraging stasis.

De-stitching

This should be on the fifth day, and when the stitches are removed the incisions are protected by the application of Steri-strip dressings.

The pressure bandages, if possible, should be left for three weeks undisturbed, by which time — with the protection of the ties — the segments should need only a support dressing.

Once the original back pressure has been removed with a tie, any residual veins can be quite simply injected (see under Vein injection), and compressed. However, the combination of well-sited local ties and compression, as described, does enable long segments of vein to be obliterated in a cosmetically acceptable way, in a relatively short time, with the danger of extraversation of the injection — with its attendant problems of discomfort, fat necrosis and patient unhappiness — very much reduced. It also diminishes the chance of getting the long segment of vein thrombosed with injection with the blood still in it, leading to a disfiguring brown staining following resolution of the phlebitis so caused, which also causes the same end result for the patient.

However, the surgeon is subjecting the patient to a scar on the leg, but it is considered that if this is sited well and is small it is usually much more cosmetically acceptable than the just-mentioned hazards of injection of large varicosities.

★ ★ ★

Venous flares

The treatment of venous flares has proven very difficult and is still very unsatisfactory.

Spidery venous flares are due to distended capillaries and venules, which are actually in the skin itself and not lying underneath it. They cause marked cosmetic embarrassment, but are no other danger apart from this.

Injection of these flares is technically very difficult indeed and, if normal sclerosant is used, is fraught with hazard and disaster as the skin overlying the flare — even if the injection has been satisfactory — does tend to slough. In the best cases this results in linear scarring, and, in the worst cases, quite a substantial skin loss.

It is very strange in fact that quite often patients at the end of the day prefer to have the white scarring rather than the cosmetically difficult-to-hide flare itself.

Attempts have been made to inject these flares using magnifying glasses and microneedles with hypertonic saline and also with hypertonic sugar solutions. Although at the time of the injection, if it is successful from its feeding vein, the flare does blanch and it seems that the surgeon has obtained a very good result, at the end of the day the long-term results are very poor.

Overall, an attempt to inject these venous flares should not be undertaken.

However, the flare is fed by a single venule and can be controlled by pressure on that feeding site so logically one should be able to improve the situation.

The best results are obtained by attempting to thrombose the feeding vein using an electrolysis needle similar to the instrument used for the elctrolysis of unwanted hair. This is a very fine electrode introduced along the hair follicle and then when in place the electrolysis is carried out destroying the hair root.

This has been used with success for the treatment of venous flares and indeed at the end of the day the surgeon has an enormously satisfied patient, but even with this seemingly simple procedure it is very difficult to get thrombosis.

★ ★ ★

Toe-nail surgery

Removal of toe-nail

Indications

1. As the first preliminary stage in the treatment of a grossly ingrowing toenail.
2. For some cases of chronic paronychia.
3. For acute paronychia to facilitate drainage.
4. Relating to trauma where the nail has been damaged or partially avulsed already.
5. First stage of nail-bed ablation or wedge excision of nail-bed.

Special documentation

The digit must be specified in all notes by its side fully written and the digit in question identified as described before, and this must be checked with the patient before the operation.

Shaving

Not really necessary unless there are a few hairs lying on the dorsum of the toe which need removing.

Surgical anatomy

The nail lies on its nail-bed formed from the underlying very vascular connected tissue which gives it its pink colour, with the exception of that area at the proximal end near the root of the nail called the lunula or moon which is white and appears more opaque due to the underlying area being not so vascular.

The nail grows from the proximal end or root of the nail from the zona germinative or deeper layer of the epidermis.

The superficial layer of the epidermis or zona cornea of the skin surrounding the nail stops at the proximal end of the nail where it folds back and is attached to the superficial surface of the underlying nail to form a thin cuticular fold or eponychium. Distally at the free edge of the nail this layer starts again on the under-surface of the nail to which it is attached and is then continuous with the zona cornea of the skin of the digit tip.

Laterally the nail is overlapped by a fold of the zona cornea called the lateral nail fold which is continuous with the eponychium proximally.

Nail growth

The nail grows at its root at its proximal end from the zona germinative and becomes thicker under the lunula and is gradually pushed forward from this growing area.

The orderly arrangement in this area can be disturbed leading to abnormal nail growth in conditions such as:

1. Onychogryphosis.
2. Related to trauma.
3. Ingrowing toenail.

Instruments

A standard setting

Additional instruments
Digital rubber tourniquet
Two Kochers artery forceps

Dressings

Steri-spon or Oxycel haemostatic
absorbable sponge dressing
Steristrip skin closures

Position on table

With pathology in the nail of a digit of the foot the patient is lying flat on his back on the table. For operation and removal of the nail of the finger the patient should be on the table, as before, lying comfortably but the arm and hand should be out at the side on a separate table or trolley to facilitate ease of access.

Area of sterile field

The whole hand up to the wrist or the foot from the forefoot down to the toes, should be cleansed with skin preparation and, having put the cleansed limb down onto a sterile towel, a further towel is then laid over and wrapped round the wrist or forefoot, isolating the surgical field without having towels intruding and cutting down the operating exposure. It is best to use the general purpose trolley towels rather than one with a hole in it.

Paintup

It is very important, as the surgeon is going to use a tourniquet, that the paintup is not heavily coloured as, post-operatively any colouration of the skin which remains makes it difficult to assess the return of the blood supply following the removal of the tourniquet.

Anaesthesia

Surgical block is established (as described in Chapter 6), using 2% Lignocaine without Adrenalin. Adrenalin should *never*, repeat *never*, be used under any circumstances in a digit, whether a tourniquet is used or not.

Application of a tourniquet

This makes precise dissection much easier and a perfectly adequate tourniquet is provided by a soft rubber tube which is put round the root of the digit in the area of the digital block, and then stretched and clipped in that position by a strong artery forcep, such as a Kochers.

When clipping the rubber, great care should be taken that a fold of underlying skin is not included in the clamp because if it is, this causes more post-operative pain and discomfort than the rest of the operation put together. The tourniquet and clamp should, at all times, be visible and never hidden under the towels (Figure 12.4).

Figure 12.4 Application of a tourniquet

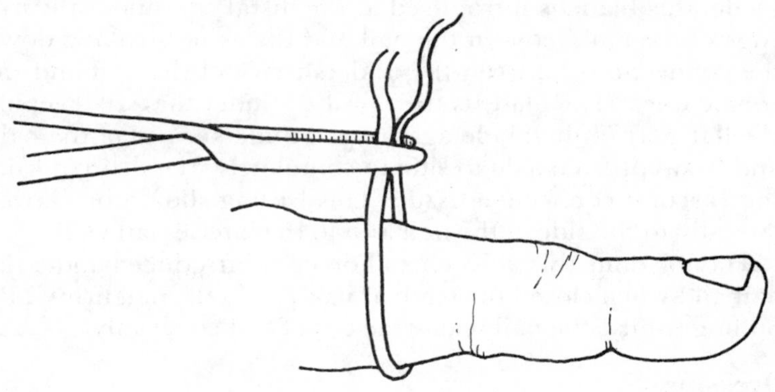

Surgical technique

Any operation on a hand or digit is a precise surgical procedure and in no way must it become a quick snatch and avulsion of a nail in a few minutes' rushed procedure at the end of a list.

If it is carried out carefully with due regard to the anatomy, the nail will grow again in its normal true elegant shape, given no underlying pathology, and its growth will not be distorted by bad surgery.

The nail may grow out repeating the abnormaility for which surgery has been undertaken, such as an ingrowing toenail or onychogryphosis, but the abnormality will not be one that has been created by barbaric surgery.

As can be seen by the anatomy, in order to free the nail and remove it, the zona cornea of the skin over the nail-bed, where it is reflected onto the nail at the eponychium, has got to be divided and not just avulsed. The undersurface of the nail has got to be freed from the underlying vascular connective tissue, and the undersurface of the nail at the distal border near its free edge has got to be once again divided from the zona cornea just as at the eponychium.

Having established local anaesthetic with a tourniquet, the digit is held with the left hand and with a 15 blade the eponychium is formally cut across the base of the nail separating the attachment of the skin to the dorsal part of the nail.

A large artery forcep is then taken and opened and using one blade, this blade is introduced at the distal end under the free edge of the nail between the nail and the skin, breaking down the connections between the undersurface of the nail and the zona cornea. The blade is then pushed under the nail, keeping the flat part of the blade against the undersurface of the nail, and is swept from side to side to completely free the nail from the vascular connective tissue. This freeing should be carried laterally to the side of the nail and to the lateral nail wall.

Having done this, a Kochers Forcep is introduced under the nail and when closed the teeth at its tip grip the nail firmly. By pulling firmly, the nail will come out of its bed cleanly.

Dressings

At this stage the nail-bed, although vascular, should not — due to the tourniquet — be bleeding. An oxycel or other haemostatic absorbable sponge dressing should be placed over the nail-bed and packed firmly into the lateral fold where the nail has been removed and also under the proximal skin flap where the eponychium has been divided.

This oxycel is then held in place by two or three Steristrip dressings going from one side to the other, but not completely encircling the pulp of the digit.

The combination of the firm pressure applied by the Steristrip dressings and also the effect of the haemostatic sponge means that further dressings put on top of the digit can the next day be removed, leaving the lower Steristrip dressing undisturbed for two or three days, after which it can be soaked off with some Savlon or half-strength Eusol.

At all times with the dressings, the skin of the terminal part of the pulp of the digit must be visible and the whole digit must never be covered completely from sight.

Before the final dressings are put on, the tourniquet is removed and the skin of the pulp of the digit is inspected to ensure that the capillary blood supply has returned.

Post-operative care

The patient is advised to rest the foot as much as is possible for the first 48 hours with the foot elevated to try to diminish oedema.

The outer dressing, if soiled, can be removed and changed but the deep Steristrip dressing should not be touched if at all possible, for three days. At this time the foot can be put in warm water or a mild antiseptic solution, and the Steristrip soaked and eased off.

This may then remove some of the clot, debris and remains of the oxycel haemostatic sponge from the cavities in the lateral side of the nail-bed, revealing clean and granulating tissue.

A light dressing with a non-stick surface is then applied over the whole nail-bed and lateral cavities to try to get the area clean by letting the air get to it rather than having a totally occlusive dressing.

Whenever the toe is rinsed in warm water or a mild antiseptic solution thereafter, it should be dried and have this light non-stick dressing applied as long as is necessary for comfort or protection whilst the nail regrows from the lacuna.

★ ★ ★

Acute subungual haematoma

The important differential diagnosis here is that of a subungual melanoma which, if suspected, should always be referred on as an urgency without any attempt made at establishing the diagnosis.

The surgeon who is carrying out the definitive treatment should have all the options open to him from the start.

The subungual haematoma is an acutely painful subungual collection of blood relating to recent trauma. The haematoma eventually causes the loss of the nail which then has to grow out slowly, but in the meantime the discomfort is not inconsiderable and is also prolonged.

With trauma to the finger there is always the possibility that there may be an associated fracture of the terminal phalanx so x-rays should be carried out immediately.

If this x-ray shows a fracture then the following treatment must not be considered, and the treatment should be conservative with analgesics, etc.

If there is no fracture and a large subungual haematoma is causing considerable pain, then relief from the symptoms can be obtained in the following way.

1. Clean the finger with a water-based skin preparation, not a spirit-based one.
2. Open out a normal paper clip (Figure 12.5).
3. Grasp the loop of the clip with a pair of strong artery forceps.
4. Put the straight end into a flame from whatever source available until it is red hot.
5. Gently press the red-hot end on to the nail at right angles over the centre of the subungual haematoma.

Figure 12.5 Opened paper clip being held in flame

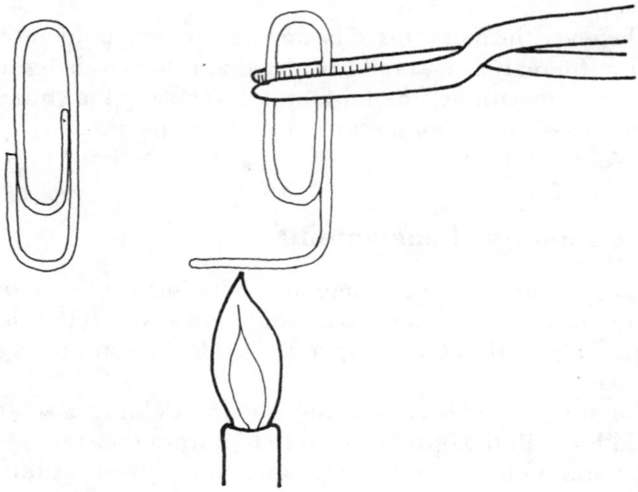

If this site is peripheral in the nail it will not need any anaesthetic as long as the pressure is not too hard, which will cause the underlying tense haematoma to become more painful.

If the site is near the 'moon' it may be sensitive despite the fact that there is a subungual haematoma related to it. If this is so the whole situation must be re-assessed at this point to see if the symptoms warrant a formal ring block of the finger being carried out, with the procedure being done under anaesthetic.

Assuming it is peripheral, gentle pressure and reheating of the pin slowly burns a hole through the nail and into the cavity of the haematoma. There will be a sudden loss of resistance as it goes through.

On withdrawal of the pin the tense blood is released, the pain is eased and dry dressings are applied.

If there is a fracture then this procedure technically converts it from being a simple fracture to a compound one and therefore should not be carried out.

Post-operatively

The nail will separate in due course as the procedure just described is one only for easing symptoms, although relieving the tension in the haematoma does perhaps slow down any further damage that it does.

In time the new nail starts to grow and push out the old nail. At this stage there is a quite considerable risk that one of the projecting sides or spikes of the old nail will be snagged or caught causing it to be partly avulsed. This is, in fact, an understandably very painful procedure, so depending on the occupation of the patient he should be seen again. At this time a decision can be made on whether it might be better to bring him up as a formal procedure. Under a ring block, a formal removal of the distal partly avulsed nail can be done so removing it from this hazard and giving the growing nail freedom to grow out unimpeded.

★ ★ ★

Ablation of toe-nail bed

The procedure is designed to stop further growth of the nail in its entirety.

Indications

Onychogryphosis is a condition usually occurring in the elderly due to alteration in the blood supply to the nail-bed. The nail becomes very hyperkeratotic and protrudes rather like a claw and is thereby in very great danger of being accidentally avulsed or causing tenderness and pain due to its protrusion when shoes are worn. In view of the underlying pathology and age group, no tourniquet should be used when ablating the nail-bed for this condition.

Occasionally the full nail-bed is ablated when past attempts at carrying out wedge excisions for ingrowing toenails have failed and the condition keeps on recurring.

Surgical technique

The first part of the procedure is as described for the removal of a toenail, with the exception that no tourniquet is used.

Once the nail has been removed, the object then is to remove all the nail generating area. Initially two longitudinal incisions are made down to the proximal angle of the nail-bed on each side and the flap of skin so formed is lifted up.

As can be seen from Figure 12.6 the incisions are made slightly diagonally which improves the access to the nail-bed in each lateral corner.

Figure 12.6 Incisions giving good access to toe-nail bed

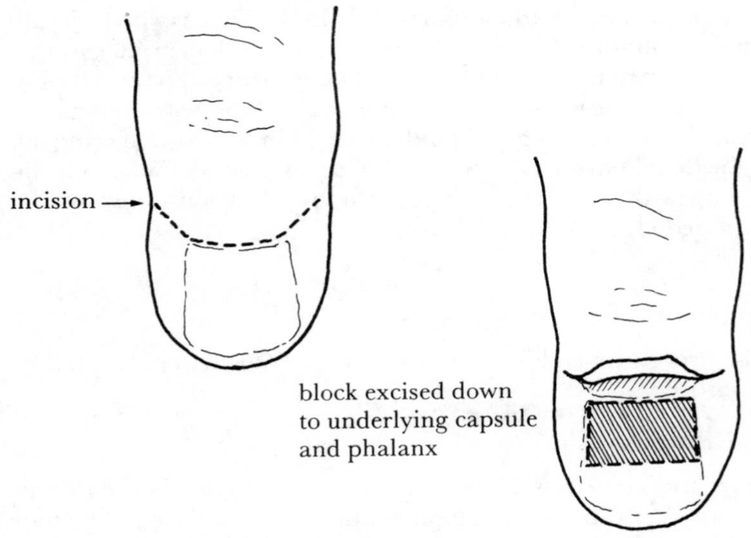

A transverse incision is now made approximately one third of the way along the nail-bed and this incision is taken down to the phalanx anteriorly and at each side.

The flap of skin is now reflected backwards with a skin hook, and a similar transverse incision is made down to the capsule of the interphalangeal joint by dissecting between the skin and white epychondrium.

These incisions are joined by lateral incisions, as seen in Figure 12.6.

The aim and object is to remove the enclosed block of tissue down to the phalanx and from the phalanx on to the capsule of the joint and laterally all the way up where the reflection of the epicondrium can be seen at its apex.

It is very important to get the lateral extensions of the nail-growing area on each side totally removed. Leaving any islets of tissue behind results in an uncomfortable spike of bone eventually developing which has to be subsequently removed as a second procedure.

Once this block of tissue has carefully been dissected out it is replaced by packing with oxycel gauze or Sterispon and the flap of skin is put back on top and held in place by a Steristrip dressing going from the side of the toe, over the flap and down to the other side.

No stitches should be used, and dressings tight enough only to control bleeding should be put on as the circulation in onychogryphosis is suspect and should not be put under threat.

Dressings placed on top of the Steristrip or Surgicell dressings should be of the non-adhesive variety so that post-operatively on the second or third day these dressings can be removed if soiled, and they will come off not bringing the underlying Surgicell dressing and clot off with it.

After four or five days the deeper dressings can be removed by cleansing with half-strength Eusol and at this time granulation should be developing and the whole area can then be dressed with non-adhesive dressings to allow the air to get to it.

★ ★ ★

Lateral nail-bed ablation

This is the surgical procedure used for the radical cure of a symptomatic ingrowing toenail.

Clinical condition

It is a condition where the sides of the big toenail begin to hook in, in a longitudinal plane, enclosing a piece of the pulp of the toe and the underlying connective tissue.

As the nail grows it digs in, this being made worse by pressure on the pulp with walking or on the nail from a shoe.

The nail wall on each lateral side being very deep, with the end of the nail digging into the tissue, causes an abscess and excessive granulomatous formation which then extrudes over the lateral side of the nail on each side.

These abscesses are probably initially started by the patient, usually in their teens, trying to trim the nail by digging down into the 'quick' on each side with the points of the scissors, rather than correctly trimming the nail.

The etiology of the condition is a little uncertain as although tight shoes, hot climate and recurrent trauma are often implicated, it has been known for ingrowing toenails to develop in a patient confined to bed for nine months with no weight-bearing at all.

Once the nail has started to grow in this way, even if it is removed and allowed to grow again, it once again grows out with the same configuration.

Initially an ingrowing toenail should be treated conservatively by:

1. *Correct trimming of the nail*
   This must be transverse or concave but not the normal convex way that a thumb nail is trimmed.
2. *Local antibiotics*
   These have no place in the treatment of this condition.
3. *Systemic antibiotics*
   (a) Associated cellulitis or a spreading infection in the toe, or,
   (b) If a foreign body, i.e. the nail, has been removed and the granulations of the abscess have been curetted out, a course of antibiotics at that stage helps to resolve the pathology.
4. *Packing under the nail*
   Packing the lateral side with cotton wool has been advocated but the long-term results have been disappointing.
5. *Treating of the granulations with silver nitrate*
   Is a very good local treatment but does not treat the underlying cause although it makes the toe very much more cosmetically acceptable.

Indications for surgical treatment

If conservative measures, conscientiously tried, have failed and the recurring pain and infection cannot be controlled.

This is a two-stage procedure:

Stage 1. Removal of the nail, as described earlier.

Stage 2. Lateral wedge excision of the nail-bed.

First-stage operation

It should be explained to the patient that in order to get the infection, abscess and granulations dealt with and the bed healed, the nail must be removed.

Following this, with the help of antibiotics — if there is any cellulitis — and dressings, the nail-bed and pulp heals and when the nail itself has started to regrow the second stage of the operation is carried out. This is done when the nail has grown out about half way and before the edges of the nail start to turn in again — usually about six weeks later.

Second-stage operation

The aim is to remove the nail-bed on each side of the root of the nail, leaving the lanula and the central half of the nail-bed untouched.

Thus, the area removed is the growing part of the nail-bed from which the nail segment, which is turning under, originates.

The middle half of the nail which is then left with the lanula, grows out flat and although it does not have the characteristics of a completely normal nail it is, nevertheless, cosmetically acceptable; much more so than if the nail-bed is ablated completely as is sometimes carried out.

Surgical technique

Stage 1

This is exactly the same as previously described for the removal of the nail but, additionally, the following points should be noted.

1. If there is a widespread cellulitis or infection due to the ingrowing toe-nail, a tourniquet should not be used and a

wide-spectrum antibiotic should be exhibited starting a five-day course of antibiotic one day pre-operatively, if possible.

2. As the nail at one or both sides may be affected with abscess formation and excessive granulation tissues, after the nail has been removed the abscess cavity should be curetted out before packing with haemostatic sponge.
3. The post-operative dressings, etc., are the same although if infection is present the Steristrip dressings may have to be removed earlier, and soaks in an antiseptic solution carried out more frequently.

Stage 2

This is carried out when:

1. The infection has been totally cleared up and the nail-bed is dry and healed.
2. The nail has grown out to about half its normal length, which is approximately six weeks after the Stage 1 operation.

The object of the operation is to remove the lateral half of the growing part of the nail on the side or on the sides which have previously been ingrowing, at a stage when the infection has been cleared and the ingrowing element of the nail's growth has not started to cause recurring trouble.

Special documentation for Stage 2

As the nail is clean and growing out apparently normally, it is vital to have documented which side of the tie the nail was ingrowing before the Stage 1 operation was done.

This must be written in full and described as medial or lateral side, or inner or outer side, but the side of the nail which was ingrowing must be established and documented with no abbreviations such as L or R which could be misinterpreted.

Shaving

Not needed.

Surgical anatomy

As described under removal of toe-nail (see Figure 12.6) except the surgical anatomy relating to the second stage the nail has grown out for only half its length.

Instruments, Position on table, Anaesthesia

All as previously described.

Surgical technique

As has been stressed before, the procedure for the removal of the lateral part of the nail-bed is a very precise and exact one which, if done properly, brings about incredible relief to the patient, but which if not completed satisfactorily results in an abnormal bony spike growing in the place where the nail-bed used to be and that, in itself, causes more problems.

The junction of the epicondrium with the surface of the nail is cut very precisely (as described earlier for removal of the nail), and the new half nail which has regrown is then removed by freeing deeply with one blade of an artery forcep sliding underneath the nail between the nail-bed and the undersurface of the nail, and being swept around. Once this is removed this then leaves the white thickened layer of epicondrium folded over, where the nail has been removed.

Two lateral skin incisions are now made from the proximal corners upwards and slightly laterally, as described in the total removal of the nail-bed, and the flap of skin enclosed between the two and lying anteriorly to the epicondrium is gently lifted. The epicondrial fold is now incised longitudinally in a line approximately one-third across the nail, i.e. if a bilateral wedge excision of the nail is being carried out one-third would be removed lateral to these incisions on each side and the remaining part in the middle would be the other third of the nail-bed.

The longitudinal incision is taken as high or proximal as the reflection of the epicondrium and is taken deeply down at the proximal end to the capsule of the joint and distally down on to the phalanx of the toe. The incision is then carried round laterally to include the epicondrium on the lateral reflection of the nail and meets the distal end of the original incision about two-thirds down the nail-bed.

The wedge of tissue, which is all the lateral growing part of the nail-bed, is then removed down to the bone and the capsule and the block of tissue that is removed is replaced with tightly packed Sterispon or Surgicel haemostatic sponge (Figure 12.7).

Figure 12.7 Lateral segments removed and packed with haemostatic sponge

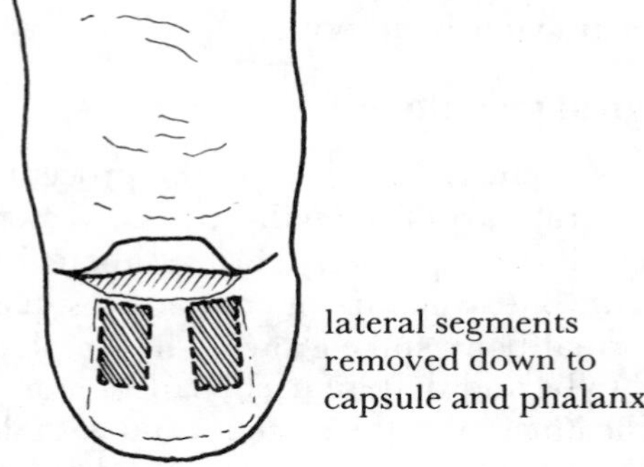

If the nail-bed has been ingrowing on both sides then a similar procedure must be done on the other side. If not, the proximal flap of skin is held in place over the packed Surgicel or Sterispon dressing with a Steristrip dressing and on top of this is placed a further layer of haemostatic sponge and then a non-adhesive dressing. It is at this stage that the tourniquet is removed so that the requisite pressure can be exerted on the dressings with the crepe bandage to control any bleeding.

The essential part of the operation is to ensure that the total white layer of epicondrium is removed intact, especially at its apex which during removal is very easy to transect and leave *in situ*.

After the operation the specimen must be examined to ensure that there is no daylight showing through the apex of the cone.

Post-operative

The top dressings are removed after 48 hours and replaced with clean ones, but if possible the Steristrip dressing and haemostatic sponge are best left, and only after another 48 hours can daily soaks with half strength Eusol be started to clean up the granulation tissue.

★ ★ ★

Local excisions

Local excision of a lipoma

The symptoms of a lipoma are usually caused by:

(a) Its size,
(b) Its cosmetic unacceptability,
(c) The fear of the patient that it is a malignant tumour.

The surgical anatomy

A lipoma is a well encapsulated, benign, fatty tumour which can occur in a slowly growing lump in either subcutaneous fat or intramuscularly.

Specific pre-operative treatment

The first priority is to re-assure the patient of the benign nature of the tumour.

Note should be specifically made of its size as it is very useful at operation to be able to refer to this if there is any doubt whether a loculus has been left behind and not dissected out.

Although the full extent of the lipoma is very obvious when first examined, this delineation can be obscured at operation by the effect of the local infiltration of the local anaesthetic.

Lights and position on the table

This depends on the site of the lesion.

Instruments

Routine general set.

Anaesthetic

Local infiltration around the tumour as has been described, but keeping an area between the tumour and the infiltration if, at all possible, clear of the infiltration so that the outer limit of the lipoma capsule can always be felt.

Although this is something to be aimed at it is very difficult to achieve in practice.

Operative technique

Incision

(a) Site. This is usually made directly over the tumour as a single incision in the line of election. However, if the tumour has been enlarging over the years and has been growing in the subcutaneous layer, it may be protruding the skin and becoming pedunculated. In this case the redundant skin has to be removed by an elliptical incision with its central line centred along the line of choice.

(b) The extent of the incision depends on the depth of the lipoma. If it is superficial an incision over it extending for half of its diameter will usually suffice. If, however, it is deeper, then in order to obtain access the incision may have to be equal to or slightly longer than the diameter.

Having cut through the skin, the subcutaneous tissue is cut in the same line with the small knife blade — round-pointed is best — until the smooth surface of the lipoma capsule is reached.

The subcutaneous tissue is locculated with fibrous tissue strands and the capsule is smooth and of a more definite homogenous appearance. Although both have fatty contents, they are markedly different. This can be seen with experience.

Having reached the capsule, the lateral dissection over the lipoma surface is carried out on each side. Initially the skin and any fat leading down to it is everted by holding with a Mayo forcep and the plane demonstrated is cleaned with a knife by using the blade upside down, i.e. with the sharp edge of the blade facing superficially, not deeply to the capsule.

If this is gently swept around the plane between the capsule and the subcutaneous fat, this separates the plane very satisfactorily.

At this stage the capsule of the lipoma can be grasped with the *Mayo forcep*. It is a dangerous practice to get hold of this with an artery forcep, or with a tissue forcep, as both of these instruments can tear the capsule of the lipoma when they are being pulled upon to give traction. Once the capsule is torn it makes the subsequent dissection very much more difficult.

The dissection is continued and carried on by the use of fine scissors or an artery forcep that is introduced in the shut position into the plane which has already been developed, then opened up separating the plane even more, any strands being cut with the scissors.

The separation should be done progressively with each side and the ends being at about the same amount of progress all the time. In this way it presents in the incision much more easily than trying to dissect one side completely before starting on the other.

This dissection is continued until the tumour is virtually free. At this stage there may be a core of connective tissue with an odd small vessel running in it coming into the deep surface. If this presents well it can be clipped with an artery forcep, the tumour separated proximately, and the vessel tied with a fine 40 plain catgut tie.

Usually the tumour comes out and any bleeding is controlled by a few moments pressure.

The cavity from which it has come now has to be closed.

Following the removal it does tend to fall in a little, and usually a little deep mobilisation has to be carried out before the sides, which have been compressed over the years, come together without tension.

This cavity is then closed with deep catgut stitches. These stitches are best put in with a curved, round-bodied needle and, depending on the size of the cavity, if some of the stitches can be put in upside down, as described earlier, with the knots buried, it makes the post-operative problems less likely.

Skin stitches

If there has been adequate deep closure, a through-and-through stitch at a maximum of 5 mm separation can be used, or if there is absolute certainty of the deep closure, an intracutaneous fine nylon stitch can be used.

Probably the best stitch for this sort of procedure is either the intracutaneous or a combination closure of stitches and Steri-strips, as previously described.

Following the stitches, a non-adhesive dressing is first applied and then some form of firm, post-operative pressure dressing should be put on. This need not be too tight, but a firm dressing does cut down any possibility of deep haematoma forming.

The superficial dressing, whether it be a crepe bandage or strapping, depending upon the site, can be removed after 48 hours, leaving the Steristrip dressings and the deep dressing in place.

Removal of stitches
If a combination stitch has been used, the stitches will be removed on the fourth to fifth day, leaving the Steristrip dressings in place. New Steristrip dressings are put over the site where the skin stitches have just been removed, so that the whole incision is now supported with Steristrip for a further week.

All through-and-through stitches
If the incision has been sewn up with all through-and-through stitches, alternative stitches should be removed on the third day and these replaced with Steristrip dressings, the remaining stitches being removed on the fifth day and similarly replaced.

An intracuticular stitch
This is removed on the fifth day, but before it is removed Steristrip dressings should be placed over the incision to support it for the following few days after the subcuticular stitch has been removed.

Pathology

Despite the seemingly benign nature of the lipoma, it must always be sent for definitive histological examination.

In the future it is then never a matter of opinion as to what its nature was, but one of microscopical fact which can be shown to the patient if any worries develop later.

Intramuscular lipoma

Here the lesion is deeper. The subcutaneous tissue, as described earlier, is divided down to the fascia of the muscle which presents as a shining, silver fascial plane. The plane, if necessary, is opened up a little bit to provide access using the same technique with scissors and artery forceps.

Having confirmed that the lipoma is lying deeper, the fascia of the muscle is divided in the direction of the muscle fibres.

Great care must be taken not to divide this fascia across the muscle fibres as the danger of developing a muscle hernia afterwards is quite considerable.

The muscle, following the division of the fascia, then usually bulges through the gap due to the lipoma underneath it. The muscle fibres are then separated in a longitudinal direction over the lipoma. This does not usually produce any significant bleeding.

Once the surface of the capsule of the lipoma is reached it usually enucleates very easily and surprisingly free from any further bleeding.

Following removal, the muscle fibres fall together and can be held with a few gently applied and lightly tied catgut 40 stitches on a round-bodied, curved needle.

The muscle sheath is closed with 40 catgut stitches as once again there should be no strain on this if it has been cut in the right direction.

The rest of the procedure is as previously described.

Post-operatively, the only difference is that perhaps movement of the muscle is encouraged to stop adhesions and stiffness and spasm developing which, in themselves, cause more discomfort.

* * *

Lymph gland biopsy

A gland biopsy may well be advised to establish a diagnosis in a case of general or local regional glandular englargement, whether this is due to an infection or a tumour.

If the gland is isolated and single then the freedom of choice as to which gland to remove is not present. However, if the gland is one of a mass of glands, the decision of which gland to remove does become important.

It may be that a lump of doubtful aetiology has been removed which subsequently turns out to be a gland.

If at all possible, the whole individual englarged gland should be removed rather than trying to take a wedge or piece out of it for histological examination. This is because:

1. Control of the bleeding is easier
2. Any spread of either tumour or infection, post-operatively, must be reduced.

Surgical anatomy

The lymphatic system, arterial system, venous system and nervous system wherever in the body tend to run together.

If ever a gland is enlarged it must always be assumed that in the immediate proximity there are vessels present and that these vessels are not small capillaries associated with the blood supply of the gland itself, but are much more likely to be of a larger significant size.

The lymph gland itself, whatever its pathology, is likely to have a good vascular supply probably enhanced by its intrinsic pathology. If an artery is accidently damaged it bleeds from one end and with pressure which encourages it to go into spasm and with the bleeding reduced there is much more chance of it being able to be controlled.

If a vein is torn, the dark blood continues bleeding usually from both ends and getting control of it may be very troublesome.

If the gland which is chosen to be removed is isolated, rather than being one of a chain, it will have a capillary blood supply of its own which usually can be tied as a separate entity keeping very much more control of the whole operative field.

Therefore, the surgical anatomy of the site around the gland will vary in the specific place where it is, but the principle of the lymphatic system being one of a bundle should always be remembered.

Site of election

If a gland biopsy is to be carried out to enable a diagnosis to be established from a generalised glandular enlargement, the factors to be considered are:

1. If possible take an isolated gland rather than one of a matted chain.
2. A mobile gland is better than one that is fixed or tethered deeply.
3. Try to take a superficially placed gland rather than a deep one because (a) access is better, (b) associated vessels are probably smaller and not so significant.
4. Whether one can get a good scar in a skin crease, or a scar hidden away out of sight.

Surgical technique

Specific techniques cannot be described as the site varies. However:

1. Having decided which gland to go for pre-operatively make certain it is documented accurately and, if necessary, marked with a skin pen before infiltration with local anaesthetic.
2. Once local anaesthetic infiltration has been carried out, the palpable gland may very often disappear so the surgeon must be certain to know beforehand where and how long the incision is going to be.
3. If possible, and with a mobile gland, keep it steady between the thumb and index finger of the left hand whilst you incise the skin and subcutaneous tissue. You can then slowly progress down to it by opening and closing artery forceps or scissors, and not be liable to pass the gland by, go too deep and get into further trouble.
4. The characteristics of the gland will depend on the pathology but whatever is the pathology, it usually results in the gland being very friable.
5. When you have reached the gland gently dissect around it by opening and closing an artery forcep.
6. Do not grab the gland with an artery forcep or tissue forcep as this will inevitably squash and burst it. This leads to increased difficulty getting it out and also an increased chance of spreading cells or infection around.
7. If bleeding occurs treat with pressure. If that does not stop it, then treat with more pressure again before trying to resort to attempting to pick up with artery forceps any particular bleeder.

   There is usually potential trouble around the gland wherever it is situated and more harm can be done by impatience than ever by waiting and pressing on the site and letting nature help you.
8. Having mobilised most of the gland, if there is an adventitial bundle leading to it with vessels or a dilated lymphatic, clip and tie it with catgut under direct vision.

Remember

1. A gland in the axilla or the neck is always deeper than you think.
2. The groin has often chronic shotty glands which may not be relevant and as the infection rate in this region is probably higher, it is better to avoid this area unless there is a specific reason to try to excise a gland here, such as a secondary gland from some pathology in the leg or peri-anal region.

★ ★ ★

Mucous cyst of mouth or ranula

This mucous cyst of the floor of the mouth, or sometimes even going on to the lip, presents as a painless swelling which is causing trouble with eating, or perhaps causing cosmetic embarrassment as it can grow to quite a large size.

Pathologically it is thought to be due to degeneration in a mucous gland and it is sometimes called a simple retention cyst of the floor of the mouth.

The cyst contains mucus and never salivary juices, so does not appear to be related to any of the salivary glands.

Preparation

Good dental hygiene and a mouth wash pre-operatively.

Position on table

It is usually better to have the patient in an upright position on a chair, thus if any bleeding occurs it is swallowed and not inhaled.

However, if the patient is of a nervous disposition and likely to feel faint it is better lying flat, but to have the patient on one side or the other if at all possible.

Instruments

A general set with the addition of a fine 40 catgut stitch being available.

Anaesthetic

2% Lignocaine Gel is put on a swab or cotton wool ball and put up against and held against the cyst and adjacent mucosa. This superficial anaesthesia is all that is necessary but the mucosa of the cyst and the surrounding area must be given time to become anaesthetised before surgery starts.

Operative procedure

Sterilisation of the mouth is impossible so it should not be attempted.

A small blade is stoked across the dorsum of the anaesthetised cyst.

The thickness that has to be traversed is very, very small and if there is to be any chance that the cyst is to be removed intact the depth of the incision must be equal all over the dome and the surgeon must be very, very gentle.

The cyst wall is obvious when it is revealed, but rarely is it not breached. Once the wall is reached it is separated rather like a sebaceous cyst. If by any chance it is removed intact the mucosa is left to drain, but this state of affairs is usually a rarity.

It is much more likely that in attempting to find the right layer the cyst is opened and the mucus content then discharges. If possible, at this stage, if the cyst wall can be identified and grasped with very fine artery or mosquito forceps some of it can be avulsed and removed.

Following the discharge of the mucus and the opening of the cyst through a linear incision, the opening into the dome of the cyst must now be widened by excising more of the mucosa stretched over it and the cyst wall in a wide ellipse and then the remains of the cyst is marsupralised.

Marsupralisation entails sewing the mucosa to the cyst wall with some interrupted 40 (or finer) fine catgut plain atraumatic sutures so that the cyst does not heal over once again and reform. Thereafter any discharge or mucus from the cyst goes straight into the mouth. This marsupralisation seems to be a very good definitive treatment.

As the surgeon is dealing with structures in the floor of the mouth, stitches must be placed carefully and superficially with particular reference to not under-running or involving the submandibular salivary gland duct, or any of the deeper arteries or nerves in that region. For this reason the stitches should be fairly superficial and never deep stitches trying to control bleeding, which can be perfectly well controlled by pressure if it occurs.

Post-operatively

Mouthwashes should be prescribed as necessary and quite frequently. It is always a good point to use a red or pink coloured mouthwash. This is because there is bound to be some blood or bloody discharge and it is less worrying for the patient if the mouthwash starts off the same colour as it finishes when it is spat out.

★ ★ ★

Ganglia

A ganglion is a tense cystic swelling which usually communicates either with a joint or a tendon sheath and contains a gelatenous fluid of similar consistency to synovial fluid of the joint.

Ganglia may occur in any region where a tendon or joint is situated but the most common site is the back of the hand or sometimes the dorsum of the foot.

Either of these situations is amenable to surgery under block anaesthesia as described before. This means that there is a tourniquet in place which makes the surgery very much easier.

However, it must be said that the only situation where ganglia should be attempted to be removed under local anaesthetic is on the dorsum of the hand or the dorsum of the foot.

Ganglia that occur either on the radial or ulnar border or the palmar surface of the hand, or in any other sites are not suitable for excision by those not specialised in this particular surgery. This is because the hazards of damage to surrounding vital structures in those regions are very high.

If a ganglion is to be excised on the dorsum of the hand or foot, it is advised that just as with a vasectomy the general practitioner should seek the help of his consultant orthopaedic colleague at the local hospital. He should stand in during some surgical sessions where these cases are being done. If the operation is carried out under general anaesthetic there can be free discussion of the technique and the problems.

The dissection is a very precise one and provides great satisfaction to the surgeon when it is accomplished well. However, the vital important element is being able to recognise tissue such as nerves and vessels in a field which is bloodless due to a tourniquet.

Also, as the situation of ganglia is so varied the removal of them is very difficult to describe from the anatomical point of view as the anatomy of the peripheral nerves, tendons, tendon sheaths etc., will be totally different depending on from where the ganglia are originating.

Therefore, in summary, although this surgery is suitable for carrying out in those controlled situations in a general practice surgical environment, it should be done only in those cases on the dorsum of the hand and on the dorsum of the foot and only after having been involved in instruction with a local consultant.

★ ★ ★

Surgery of bursae

Olecranon bursa

Indications for removal are related to:

1. The unacceptable cosmetic appearance of the lump.
2. A history of recurrence after trial aspiration.
3. A history of infection previously treated by antibiotics, with or without drainage.

Documentation

Once again the importance must be stressed of accurately documenting the size and side where the bursa was first seen as the size may have since varied.

Shaving

If the arm is hairy it is better to shave about 8 cm above and below the elbow.

This is not only for the sake of sepsis, but it also makes the application of strapping and its subsequent removal very much easier.

Surgical anatomy

The bursa lies over the olecranon of the ulnar but is always superficial to the deep fascia. It may be adherent and very stuck to the undersurface of the skin.

There is no communication with the joint. The bursa can be removed intact and the deep fascia should not be breached.

Instruments

A general set.

Position on the table

This is one of personal choice, but having the patient lying face down on the table with the arm out at a right angle on an arm-support, medially rotated, brings the ulnar facing upwards. This is probably the most comfortable for the patient and easiest for the surgeon.

Anaesthetic

Local infiltration, remembering:

1. The ulnar nerve runs in the groove behind the medial epicondyle of the humerus and then lower lying on the medial side of the medial ligament of the elbow joint. It is at this point that it should be palpated and identified before infiltrating the subcutaneous area around the bursa so that accidental involvement of the nerve does not occur.
2. Keep all the infiltration superficial to the deep fascia.

Technique

Following infiltration, a longitudinal incision made directly over the bursa through the skin comes right down on the surface of the bursa capsule.

Having reached the fibrous capsule it has to be dissected out actively with a small-bladed knife, preferably without a point.

Once the planes are developed it comes to hand progressively more easily.

The bursa itself can be grasped with Mayo or Russian forceps and the skin edges retracted with skin hooks or a small self-retaining retractor to provide better access.

Direct cutting dissection is very much better, particularly in the early stages where the bursa has to be separated from skin, than using or trying to use blunt dissection with a swab.

Pressure is usually sufficient to control any oozing.

Interrupted through-and-through skin stitches supported by Steristrip straps between them should be used if the area is dry at the end of the operation. This should be then followed by a gauze dressing with a generous wad of cotton wool on top followed by a firm crepe bandage to provide a firm and evenly spread pressure which is not going to obstruct the limb distally.

If there is oozing which does not stop, a small glove drain may be left *in situ* which comes out at one end of the incision.

This should be carefully recorded in the notes and there should be a generous dressing over it to allow any seepage to be soaked up.

The drain should be removed after 24 hours and a new, firm crepe bandage applied afterwards.

De-stitching — should occur on the fifth or sixth day after which firm dressings should be re-applied for a further few days.

Post-operative movement is encouraged within the restrictions that are present from the crepe bandage.

★ ★ ★

Infra-patella bursa

Although there is a small bursa called the deep infra-patella bursa which lies deep to the ligamentum patellae, the usual infra-patella bursa is that which is also called Housemaid's knee, when it is enlarged.

It lies subcutaneously between the skin and the deep fascia and the indications for removal are the same as for the olecranon bursa.

Surgical anatomy

The bursa lies subcutaneously between the skin and the insertion of the patella tendon into the tibial tuberosity.

It is totally superficial to the deep fascia and does not communicate with the joint.

Instruments

A general set.

Position on the table

The patient is best lying flat on his back on the table.

Anaesthetic

Local infiltration subcutaneously around the bursa.

Surgical technique

A transverse incision is made over the bursa coming down immediately onto the capsule. This is then dissected out with the same technique as that used and previously described for the olecranon bursa.

It should be emphasised that a sharp knife dissection, particularly in the early stages of the removal, is very much more preferable to trying to get the layers developed with blunt dissection with a swab.

Stitching and post-operative management are the same as with the olecranon bursa.

★ ★ ★

Pre-patella bursa

The subcutaneous pre-patella bursa lies between the lower part of the patella and the skin. Only on occasions when it is very large can it be confused with the supra-patella bursa.

The differentiation between these two is important as the supra-patella bursa does communicate with the joint, whereas the subcutaneous pre-patella bursa lies between the patella and the skin and has no deep communication.

Surgical anatomy

The infra-patella branch of the saphenous nerve sweeps round from the medial side of the knee joint running downwards and laterally around in front of the patella. It supplies the area below the patella with its sensory nerve supply.

This cutaneous nerve is liable to damage so its position should be recognised and it should be looked out for as the dissection proceeds.

Surgical technique

A transverse incision over the pre-patella bursa heals well and minimises the chance of damage to the nerve.

Once the capsule is reached, as long as the dissection keeps close to the capsule while it is being removed and as long as the dissection is sharp and not blunt using a swab which might damage surrounding tissues, the risk of damage to the nerve is reduced.

Once the bursa has been removed, the post-operative stitching, management and treatment is the same as previously described for olecranon bursa.

* * *

Trauma

Patients suffering major trauma resulting from a road traffic accident, or a serious accident in the home, tend to go immediately to the local hospital casualty department or accident centre. Patients with minimum trauma usually prefer more immediate treatment by their general practitioner, particularly if it is known that the facilities and expertise are available in the surgery.

For convenience of description the topic can be seen under:

1. Incisive clean trauma,
2. Incisive dirty trauma,
3. Problems of associated pathology,
4. Crushing injuries and flaps.
5. Use of antibiotics and antitetanus

1. Incisive clean trauma

Injuries caused by knives, broken glass, or other sharp instruments result in the same kind of incision as discussed elsewhere. However, pre-operative clinical assessment of the injuries to determine if there is any associated damage to deeper structures, such as nerves or tendons, is vitally important and should be carried out diligently.

As all the clinical findings can be of paramount importance both for the immediate management and, indeed, perhaps for future litigation, it is vitally important in the documentation to ensure that all is recorded at the time when seen and not later from memory. It is good practice to record all the positives as well as negatives.

If, for example, the sensation distal to the injury is lost, that will be recorded, but it is also important that if it is found to be present that too should be recorded.

It is also very important to note accurately functional loss and areas of sensation loss.

Surgical anatomy

Variable

Instruments

General set

Position on the table

Variable

Anaesthesia

With a fresh wound it is quite often possible to carry out infiltration with local anaesthesia by inserting the needle through the incision and infiltrating subcutaneously, thus avoiding even the discomfort and apprehension caused by the injection itself.

In the majority of cases it is always worthwhile infiltrating rather than hoping that the area is still a little numb from the trauma, and telling the patient it is only a few little pricks.

In proper anaesthesia the situation is under full control. The wound can be inspected as fully as possible and as necessary and care can be taken to ensure the best possible result.

Once all is cleaned, then the wound is treated, as described earlier, with as neat a scar as possible being obtained despite its direction and siting, which may not be one of first choice.

The skin edges in an incised wound are usually clean and totally viable, so, by definition, as long as the incision which has been caused is a vertical one, it does not need trimming or other modification. However, if the incision is oblique or bedvilled and, if by converting these edges to vertical edges there is going to be no significant increase in the tension when sewing up, then this should be done as the final result will be a very much better healed scar.

Interrupted sutures — rather than a continuous intracuticular suture — should always be used as there must be an increased element of risk of infection, and a single stitch may need to be removed at a later date.

2. Incised dirty wounds

This deserves separate mention as although all the points previously made for incised wounds are relevant, it is of increasing importance to have proper anaesthesia so that an adequate time to search for and remove any foreign body, such as glass fragments or gravel, etc., can be carried out.

Also, it is important in the record of the procedure to note what has been removed and whether it was thought that a particular fragment was removed intact, or that there was the possibility of part of it remaining which could in the future cause further trouble.

If a foreign body has been removed and it is radiopaque it is perhaps wise in the post-operative period for an x-ray to be taken to reassure both surgeon and patient that there is no further fragment remaining.

The result of this x-ray should be documented in case of the possibility of any later medico-legal action in which the surgeon might be involved with reports, etc.

3. Problems of associated pathology

If associated pathology such as a nerve or tendon damage is suspected clinically before surgery is contemplated, it is better to refer the case there and then to the local accident centre or hospital. This does give the surgeon, who ultimately has the responsibility of treating these injuries, the opportunity to assess definitively the immediate situation.

If the injury is not suspected clinically but is, in fact, found once the operation is underway, then

(a) No repair of tendon or nerve should be attempted at this stage,
(b) Accurate, precise and detailed notes should be made of the extent, type and site of damage found at this procedure,
(c) The wound should be sewn up on its own merits.

Post-operatively before the patient leaves he, or she, should be informed that deeper damage is suspected and that the definitive treatment at this stage is, and has been, primary suture, and that when the initial healing has taken place, and the swelling has been reduced, it will be referred to the relevant specialist for future assessment and management, and that this will be arranged.

It should also be documented in the notes exactly what the patient has been told, and in the referral letter to the specialist this should be included with the report of the findings at the surgery.

4. **Crushing injuries and flaps**

A crushing injury, or an injury caused by a shearing force, causes tissue damage of a quite considerable degree.

The immediate dead, devitalised tissue is usually obvious. The viable areas of skin and tissue are usually obvious, but there is a considerable area of no-man's land in between these two definite areas where doubt is present.

This is also a problem area for the most skilled surgeon as well, so it is only one of degree and judgement.

All dead tissue must be removed. If it is left and used to close the wound it will not heal, will have to slough, and consequently leave a large area to granulate. This will result eventually in a very poor scar or will necessitate revision.

If too much tissue is removed thinking it to be non-viable, and in fact it might have been all right, then the wound presents difficulty with closure, and undercutting, etc., may be necessary to relieve tension, and suddenly the whole operation becomes a much more major procedure. Tissue planes in a potentially infected field are being opened and major skin loss around is a possibility.

For all these reasons if there is any significant element of crushing in the injury, which might also involve deeper tissues where the same strictures arise as for the skin, then the patient should be referred on.

There is much grief caused by taking on this type of injury under local anaesthetic and running into problems. For this reason the facilities of a general anaesthetic — and perhaps a little more expertise being available — should be sought.

Flaps

A flap can be caused by a shearing injury or an incisive wound.

Assessment

The apex of the flap is always a suspect area and, as a general rule of thumb, if the length of the flap is longer than twice the width of its base then it should be treated with suspicion and respect.

Edges

Quite often the edges of the flap and the corresponding area of skin from which it has come are not vertical and so the skin surface becomes bevilled. If this is so then the edges have to be trimmed so that they can be adequately and properly sutured.

Viability can be assessed if the amount of bleeding from the edge needs to be stimulated by gently wiping with a swab.

If possible always avoid keeping the flap turned back over itself. This makes for easier assessment of underlying damage, etc., but can put the blood supply of the flap in real jeopardy in a very short time. It is like applying a tourniquet to the flap.

Surgical procedure

After all the debridement has been carried out:

1. The first and most important stitch is the one at the apex.

   This is best described as putting in a vertical mattress stitch, but interposing between the two final elements going through the skin is the apex of the flap, the stitch passing intracuticularly through it (Figure 12.8). This stitch must be tightened with extreme care.

   It is very unusual for the flap to be deep enough also to include in it the deep transverse element of the mattress stitch.
2. Subsequent stitches going down the sides should be put in from the base towards the apex.

   By this means, if there is any shortness of the flap then skin can be borrowed progressively with each stitch up the outside edge, thus all the time reducing the tension on the suspect apical area (Figure 12.9).

Figure 12.8 First stitch at the apex

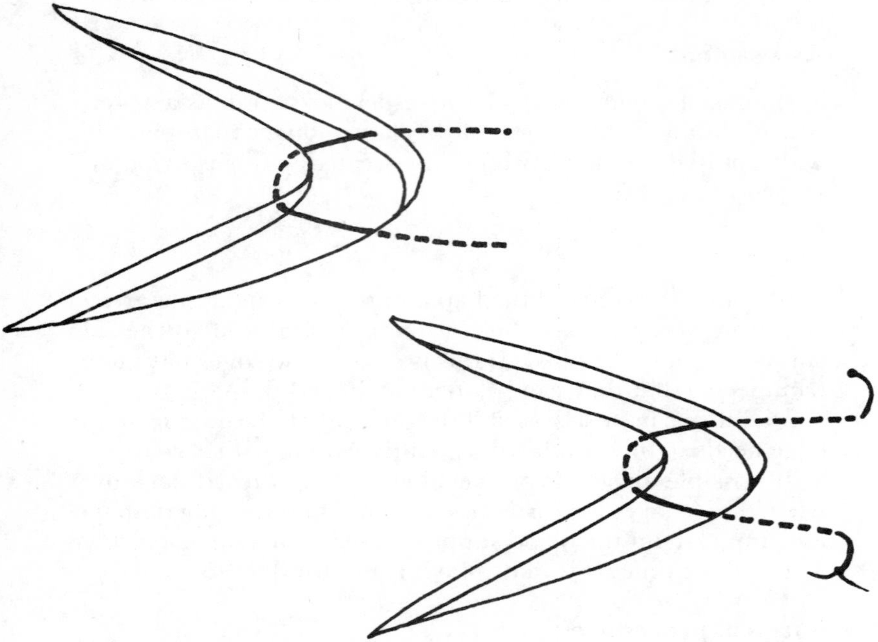

Figure 12.9 Subsequent stitches from base towards the apex

borrowing length from
the outside edge so
there is no tension
at the apex

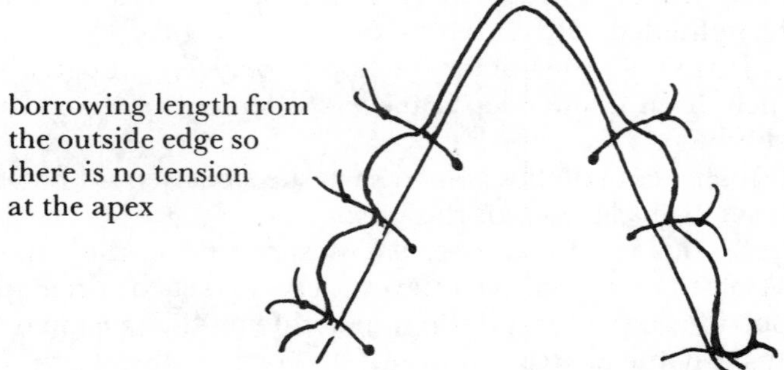

Never take the stitches too close to the apex, as by tightening up the stitches on both sides the blood supply under each stitch might be slightly impaired. Thus the only true blood supply to the actual point of the flap is that between the stitch holes on the flap itself, and this may not be enough to sustain its viability (Figure 12.10).

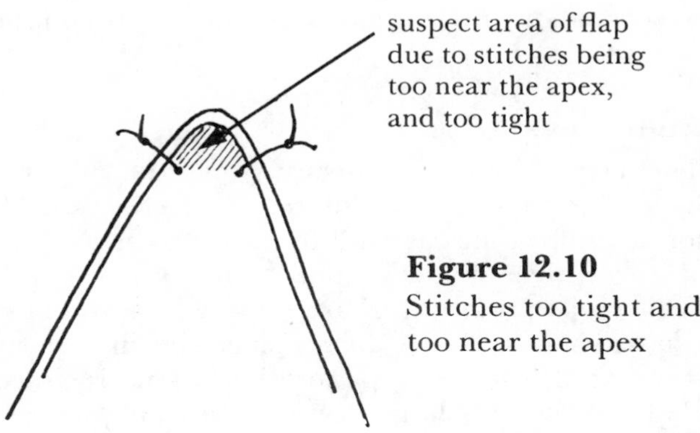

Figure 12.10
Stitches too tight and too near the apex

Although interrupted stitches do, if properly placed, tend to ease the tension on the flap, these stitches should be supplemented by judicious use of Steristrip skin straps. One strip should lead from the flap, right over its apex to the skin to try to take off the tension that way. Then, alternatively, radial straps should go over from the base of that one, outwards across the skin edge of the actual flap.

All of these are placed as indicated at the time, but the idea is not only to help skin apposition, but also to try to remove any tension from what is potentially a very suspect area.

5. **Use of antibiotics and antitetanus**

Antibiotics

When there has been trauma with the possibility of gross contamination of the wound, prophylactic use of a wide spectrum antibiotic is often indicated.

There is no substantive evidence to merit the routine use of antibiotics. However, in those cases where only a primary suture has been performed because unexpected deep complications have been encountered, indicating that secondary surgery will have to be undertaken in the near future, then it is wise to use a wide spectrum antibiotic systemically as cover.

If there is evidence of trauma associated with a compound bone fracture (often a fingertip) then it is safer, once again, to use a wide spectrum antibiotic, although there is some disagreement whether it advances healing even in such cases as these. There is never an indication for the use of a local antibiotic powder in the wound.

Antitetanus

The days of routine antitetanus cover for all types of trauma have now passed, and a more selective use is now advocated for 'tetanus prone cases'. If tetanus is to be used, the approved schedule given below should be used.

'Tetanus prone cases' are those whose wounds: have been exposed for at least 6 hours since the time of injury before being seen; are deep, perforating, or narrow-necked; or include a relatively large degree of crushing or tissue damage. Massive, clean, recent trauma does not need antitetanus cover.

Tetanus booster dose if patient already covered

0.5 ml = 40 I.U. tetanus vaccine

Tetanus dose if patient not already covered

0.5 ml = 40 I.U. stat
repeat same dose after 6 weeks
repeat same dose after 6–12 months

If the wound is large and very dirty, and possibly being referred on, the patient will need Humotet (tetanus immunoglobulin): immediate dose only, of 250 I.U.

★ ★ ★

Vasectomy

Principle of the operation

The principle is to remove a segment of the vas deferens on each side in the upper part of the scrotum thereby, as far as is possible in surgery where one is dealing with growing tissue, making it impossible for the patient to sire any further progeny.

Essential pre-operative considerations

The surgeon who is proposing to carry out this technical procedure, which it must be said at the outset is probably the most difficult one in the repertoire desribed in this book, must make some fundamental decisions regarding his own attitudes which can briefly be summarised as follows:

1. Are you prepared as the surgeon to be a pure technician? Patients seeking vasectomy will be seen by your partners in the practice as well as yourself.

   If a patient is seen by them with a request for vasectomy and the partner in question, after counselling, agrees and refers the patient to you, are you prepared to carry out the procedure on those terms?

2. If you are not prepared to be a pure technician, then you have two alternatives.

(a) To tell your partners that you consider vasectomy should be carried out only in patients within certain criteria. If they do not accept your criteria then they should refer the patient elsewhere. Otherwise, if they refer him to you, you will assume that the criteria have been upheld and that you yourself do not need to counsel the patient and his consort.

(b) To have a joint meeting and discussion with your partners regarding the criteria for vasectomy and see if you can all come to agreement as to what is acceptable and what is not.

Having reached this agreement, the points should be written down so that there is no difficulty in the future in interpretation or mistakes being made about agreed decisions.

Some of the points that obviously come up for discussion and decision in any discussion on vasectomy and about which everybody must make up their own minds are as follows:

1. Should there be a minimal age limit?

   The younger the patient the more chance there is of natural reversal and more chance, also, that there may be a request in the future for surgical reversal.

   It is important to remember that vasectomy is an operation carried out on the male, but one which is really being performed on the whole family unit, although legally a man can have a vasectomy operation performed without the consent of his wife or cohabitee. The wife, likewise, can be sterilised without the consent of her husband.

The contraceptive pill is a method of contraception which can be reversed and the younger the age group in which it is being used, the less likely it is to cause problems or side effects. For this reason some surgeons feel that in a young couple this method should be used, and the dangers of irreversible contraception pointed out to the patient. For example:

(a) Accidental loss and death of one or more of the children in the marriage. A lost child can never be replaced, but that does not alter the fact that having got over the loss, the couple may want to have another child, not to replace the lost one, but in its own right, and perhaps to be a companion for a remaining child of the marriage. This they will not be able to do following a vasectomy.

(b) The family unit may lose its mother. This loss may be due to death or formal separation and the father may then be left with small children. After having recovered from this loss, he may want to remarry and, if so, his new wife will not be able to have a child by him in their union.

It should be pointed out that the older the children are when vasectomy is carried out, the less likely it will be that the condition in the above paragraphs will be so important. For, allowing years to get over the loss of a child or a wife, the man will then be in an age bracket where to have another child by his present or new wife would not be quite so important. The earlier it is done on a patient with a young family the more exposed the family is to these risks, so a mean has to be reached where the couple use the Pill or other reversible methods of contraception in the earlier days. Then, when the family is established the man is, perhaps, more of a candidate for permanent vasectomy.

The level of this transition is obviously the point at issue when one is discussing this with one's partners.

2. The marital status and its stability and whether it should

be insisted upon that the wife should be present and fully counselled at the same time as the man for vasectomy should also be established.

3. Cohabiting status and its stability: whether the cohabitee should be involved and cognisant of the proposed vasectomy on the man.
4. Family size, etc: There is the possibility that with only a single child in the family, problems could result in a couple being left with no children. There is also the situation where there is no family and the couple at that time do not believe they ever want a family. There does seem to be a higher incidence of psychiatric problems later on in a man who has had a vasectomy and never, in fact, proved his manhood by siring any children.

The other possibility is for medical partners to agree that if a request for vasectomy arrives they do not counsel the patient themselves but refer him straight on to you as a surgeon, who then has the responsibility of counselling and the decision making of vasectomy.

If the surgeon's personal criteria for carrying out a vasectomy are not upheld, then the patient has the opportunity to go elsewhere to somebody who will perhaps be happy to perform the vasectomy.

5. A regeneration of vas and the possibility of the return of potency *must* be spelt out to the patient, even though the possibility of this happening is remote. This must always be done by whoever is the counsellor, and the partner in the practice. It must be established who is to be responsibile for explaining this to the patient and it should be the same person's responsibility to ensure the consent form is completed.

Documentation

The consent form as previously suggested does imply that the couple are counselled together, have a stable relationship and are both agreeable to the procedure being carried out.

This part may be amended if the surgeon feels happy carrying out a vasectomy on the man without his consort's knowledge or permission.

The segment which is signed by the man should not be significantly altered from the document as proposed earlier and if a surgeon feels it should be, a call to the legal department of the Medical Defence Union should be made to confirm that the surgeon is covered legally.

It must always be remembered that because of the intimate relationship of counselling a couple regarding vasectomy, there is very rarely a nurse or other person present while this discussion is going on. At the end of the day it may come down to the surgeon's own word as to what was said and explained, and how that explanation was carried on, against the combined word of the two patients relying on their memory and interpretation in a stressful situation, so always make a record on paper.

If it is felt that the consort or cohabitee or wife should be involved with the counselling and the surgeon is not prepared to do the vasectomy without that, then this documentation must be completed and consent signed by the couple together, at the same time, in the presence of the surgeon, who should countersign it at that time.

It must be explained to them that the aim is to achieve a permanent interruption of the vas on each side but because it is growing tissue there is a remote possibility that, despite all the checks carried out post-operatively to show that the operation has been done satisfactorily, that it could reconstitute itself. Although this is a remote possibility they must know that it exists.

If, however, it is felt that counselling the man is sufficient, the part of the consent form for his wife can be struck through, but the same explanation must be carried out for him.

Post-operative tests

Following explanation of the operation and the procedure, it should be emphasised to both partners that post-operative contraceptive precautions should be continued until the sperms remaining between the tie and the urethra have been washed out by multiple ejaculations. Following this, the patient should have two seminal analyses carried out at at least one week intervals which show no sperms to be present in either specimen.

The doctor should explain that he will notify the patient

when these analyses are through and under no circumstances should precautions be abandoned until that time as impregnation may occur in this post-vasectomy period.

Surgical anatomy

The vas deferens runs up from the upper pole of the epididimas and the posterior part of the spermatic cord to the external inguinal ring.

It is a thick walled 2 to 3mm diameter tube, often described as being like a piece of whipcord which can be felt through the scrotal wall.

With the vas deferens in the spermatic cord also run:

1. Arteries.
(a) Testicular.
(b) Artery to the vas which is adherent to the vas itself.

Surrounding the bundle of vas arteries and veins, etc. are layers of fascia which, from the outside in, are:

1. External spermatic fascia. This arises from the aponeurosis of the external oblique at the external ring and encloses the cord where it runs down to the testis.
2. The middle spermatic fascia or cremasteric fascia which is thicker and arises from the internal oblique muscle and contains muscle bundles of the cremasta muscle in the inguinal canal.
3. Scrotum. Composed of skin and also closely adherent to it, the Dartos muscle which is, in its turn, separated from the cord and testis by loose aerolar tissue in the scrotum.

Shaving

The scrotal skin should be shaved up to the neck of the scrotum in the groin.

If the pubic hair is long it can be trimmed but it is not necessary to shave it as the discomfort of its regrowth can then be avoided.

Instruments

1. General set with no special additions
2. Blade 15 Gillette with a short handle

3. Sutures and ties
   20 Plain catgut tie
   10 Thread of Ehticot unabsorbable tie
   30 Catgut on a curved-cutting atraumatic needle

Local anaesthetic

Usually, a pre-operative sedative should be administered. 2% Plain Lignocaine. Only 3 to 4 ml need to be drawn up but this should still be in a 20 ml syringe.

Position on the table

The patient should be flat on his back with the legs separated.

It is very important to ensure that the patient is kept, if anything, excessively warm right up to the time of the operation.

The Dartos muscle responds to cold when it retracts drawing the scrotum and testis up into a small thickened pouch. In the warm it relaxes, and the scrotal skin is thereby thin and the cord extended to its full length, and the whole operation is infinitely easier. The penis is held to the side under the upper towel so that it does not intrude on the field.

Skin preparation

Savlon which should, if possible, be warm. The normal Hibitaine in spirit should not be used as it is very painful on the scrotum, and if the Savlon is cold the Dartos contracts once again, making the whole process more difficult.

Surgical technique

This is a difficult operation to perform and it is made more difficult when it is done under local anaesthetic; it is made even more difficult still if it is done without the help of an assistant.

It is therefore recommended that, if at all possible, consultation be held with the local consultant surgeon and if the procedure is done in any of his clinics or operation sessions under a short general anaesthetic, then it is tremendously advantageous for the practice surgeon to go along and assist at the procedure.

This means to say that if the vasectomy is done under general anaesthetic, discussion, questions and answers, etc. can be carried out to a full extent without the patient being aware and made more apprehensive by such discussions taking place.

Also, the actual infiltration of the anaesthesia sometimes makes the operation more difficult and it is of immense help if the practice surgeon can assist or even carry out the operation under general anaesthetic on a few cases before starting to do it under local anaesthetic.

The help of an assistant is invaluable at certain stages of the procedure and it does need certain expertise to be able to isolate and hold the vas with one hand without an assistant being present.

In summary, one should therefore:

1. Make every effort to do a few vasectomies under general anaesthetic or at least assist at an operation under general anaesthetic before starting to do it under local anaesthetic.
2. In the early cases one should certainly have an assisant. If possible that assistant must know what is going on and know what to do at what stage without having to be instructed in front of a conscious patient under local anaesthetic.

Having painted-up and towelled-up, the whole cord is gently grasped between the thumb and index finger of the left hand through the scrotal skin at about the junction of the upper and middle third of the scrotum.

Amongst the cord the vas can be felt. The aim is to manipulate and isolate the vas from the other constituents of the cord by slowly working it and rolling it away so that eventually it feels as if the vas is lying just under the skin of the scrotum and is being held by the thumb and index finger of the left hand.

Remember that up to this point the sensitivity of the parts is still present so gentleness combined with firmness is required.

Having isolated it in this way, the assistant with the finger and thumb of her left hand, from the other side of the table, encloses the vas in the scrotal skin just lower down the scrotum and acts as counter tension to the operator's control of the upper part of the vas. This is a method whereby the vas is held so that if one end slips it is still maintained in the operative field and does not fall back into the scrotum.

Having done this, the skin between the two hands is injected with a local anaesthetic, having warned the patient beforehand that this is about to happen.

The injection is initially through the skin where the transverse skin incision is to be made, and then spreads in the subareolar tissue between the Dartos and the vas. It is not necessary, at this stage, to inject the cord itself and the total amount of injection rarely exceeds 1 to 2ml.

Having allowed time for the local anaesthetic to work, a 1cm incision is made transversely beween the two hands holding the vas and the scrotal skin. Having gone through the skin and the muscle of the Dartos, the vas can be seen under the areolar tissue which is then reached. It is a white cord-like structure enclosed in the layers of spermatic fascia.

The knife blade is then drawn gently along the length of the vas that is exposed and the external spermatic fascia and then the Middle (Cremasteric) spermatic fascia fall away leaving the white glistening surface of the vas exposed.

If sensation is still present a little local anaesthetic can be introduced alongside the vas under the fascia up and down. Remember that discomfort is not only caused by the cutting, but also by dragging down on the vas or pressure on the testis.

At this point, still maintaining the holds with the fingers, an artery forcep can be introduced under the vas between it and the fascial layers. When it is freed, which at this stage is relatively easy, it can then be bridged over the artery forcep and a Babcock tissue forcep can be put around it, thereby giving a direct hold on the vas.

It is only now that the finger holds can be released at each end by both the operator and assistant.

It is obvious how important it is to have all the instruments and ties, etc. ready within easy reach because during the first part of the operation the left hand of both the surgeon and assistant is out of action.

Having got the vas held with a Babcock tissue forcep it is then cleared up and down by gently easing off the enveloping fascial layers, which have already been divided upwards and downwards, with fine non-tooth forceps in the right hand, holding the Babcock forcep in the left and usually putting the vas itself over the index finger of the left hand to give more stability.

This is sometimes helped by further stroking the knife blade along its length both up and down from the original division of the fascial layers so that they fall back.

In amongst these layers, or sometimes still adherent to the

vas, is the artery to the vas which may need dealing with separately. Quite often it can be tied by inclusion with the first vas tie, but on occasions it is better to separate it from the vas and tie it separately. If a tie is needed the end of the fine 30 catgut can be used on a cutting atraumatic needle which is available for the skin suturing at the end of the operation.

Having cleansed and isolated about 5cms of vas it is clamped with large artery forceps, removing at least 2cms of vas between them.

Do not use fine Mosquito forceps as these sometimes tend to cut through the vas. If this happens further problems are presented as the cut end then retracts and under local anaesthetic it is difficult to recover.

This segment of vas which is removed is saved for examination microscopically later by the pathologist.

Each vas must be sent in a separate container labelled with the side and the patient's name, etc. quite clearly.

The histological report must include the fact that:

1. Both sides are examined and are confirmed microscopically to be vas.
2. The length of the vas removed is measured and documented.

The vas is then tied in the following way:

1. The forcep is held up and a 1 Ethicot or linen thread tie is put on under it. This must be tightened firmly but not too much. If it is tightened too much it might cut through the vas itself.

   The forcep is kept in position (Figure 12.11).
2. The knot is cut short and the Ethicot length in the hand is then put around the vas ¾cm along from the clip. The vas is bent over it by using the Ethicot loop against the tension of the forcep to pull up a loop of vas (see Figure 12.12). This is circled and tied with 20 catgut. Once looped over, the loop is secured by a fine Ethicot or Thread 20 tie to hold it firmly but not secured too tight, which would mean that the blood supply to the loop itself is obstructed and the loop becomes ischaemic.

   At this stage the clamp can be removed and the loop of Ethicot or Thread slipped out. The vas will retract up or down as the case may be.

Figure 12.11 Forceps kept in position

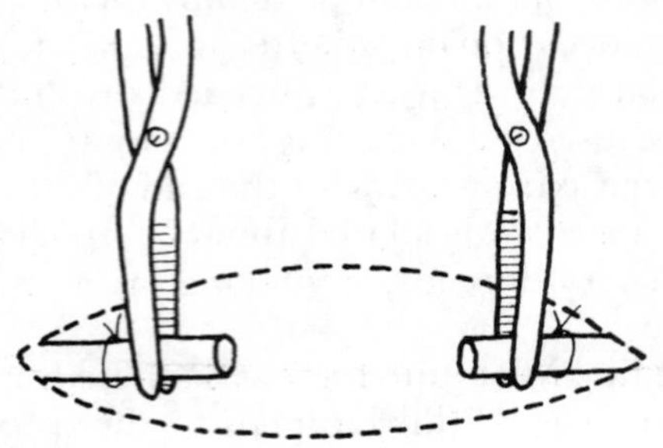

Figure 12.12 Loop of vas being pulled up

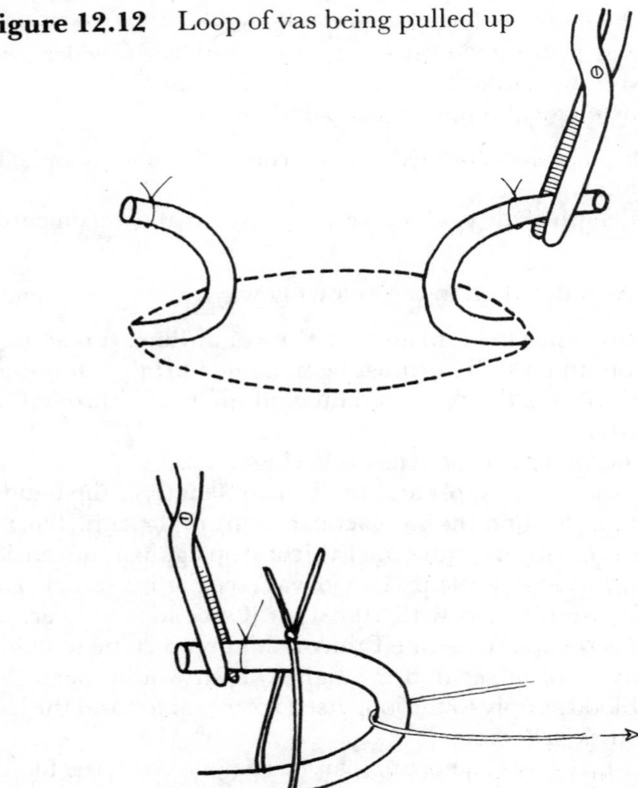

The end of the vas in the upper segment is bent over so that the ends lie inside the fascial layers that have been isolated by closing the fascial layers with interrupted 20 catgut stiches.

The end of the vas in the lower segment is bent over and an attempt is made to bury the end outside the tube of the fascial layers, thus trying to get the ends in different tissue planes.

The scrotal skin is then closed with through-and-through 30 plain catgut stitches which include the skin and the Dartos.

These stitches should be inserted so that the knots are buried. The Dartos and skin is grasped by fine forceps, turned out, and the needle is introduced from the inside. Having done this, the other side of the skin and Dartos is grasped and the needle introduced from the outside. This means that when the knot is tied it is under the Dartos and the ends of the knot do not catch on the scrotal support post-operatively.

Figure 12.13 Burying the ends of the vas in different tissue planes

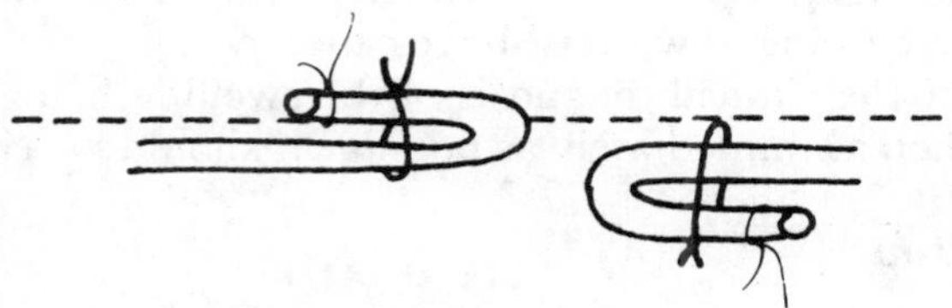

At this stage it is important once again to feel the scrotum and the vas. The two bulbous ends of the vas can be felt quite distinctly and the scrotal skin should be able to be grasped by at least a thumb's width between the ends. It is important to ensure that this gap is present when the skin is sewn up, and that the ends have not been caught up with adhesions and are lying close together.

The left vas is now resected in the same way from the same side of the table.

Having done this, a scrotal support should be worn to diminish any post-operative testicular ache. It should be worn for at least one week.

Daily baths should start 48 hours post-operatively.

After one week post-operatively, taking normal contraceptive precautions, intercourse should restart with regular ejaculation to wash out any sperms still present between the ties and the urethra.

Examination of the ejaculate should be carried out at six weeks post-operatively and two months post-operatively. It is only when two consecutive sperm counts show that no sperms are present that the patient can be notified that he may reasonably take no further contraceptive precautions.

★ ★ ★

Aspiration of cyst of breast

The aspiration of a chronic mastitic cyst or cysticfibrosis of the breast is a very simple procedure which probably brings the biggest joy and relief of all surgical procedures if assessed on a time/result basis.

The patient arrives usually distraught as either she or her husband has found a lump in the breast and from that moment on all the thoughts have been related to 'how much more life do I have remaining now that I have cancer?'

Whilst the clinical diagnosis of the swelling being cystic is made, then as immediately as possible it should be aspirated.

Aspiration

The skin is cleaned with the antiseptic of choice and the patient lying flat on her back on the table.

The cyst is enclosed between the index and thumb of the left hand and is held firmly in that position, thereby being securely fixed.

The needle on a 20 cc syringe is inserted through the skin directly into the cystic swelling.

Warn the patient there is going to be a little prick, as a sudden movement of an apprehensive patient when the prick occurs without warning sometimes makes the left hand lose control of the cyst which can then make life very difficult.

No local anaesthetic need be used, for the discomfort of putting it in is usually more than the discomfort of the aspirating needle being inserted.

The cyst is aspirated flat and the needle withdrawn.

Immediately following this the patient should be told to palpate the area and convince herself that the cyst has gone. After this, put on a cotton wool ball or a small swab over the site of the cyst to exert local pressure. Then, with the surgeon keeping the pressure on the swab in that area, the patient should replace her bra as firmly as is comfortable. The bra is pressing on the swab keeping the local pressure on the aspirated site, and the patient should wear it for at least 48 hours to try to stop the cyst reforming.

Post-operatively

1. The volume of the fluid that has been aspirated should be noted along with its characteristics of colour, etc.
2. A sample of fluid should be sent off for: (a) culture; (b) cytological examination for malignant cells.
3. The most important thing is to impress on the patient that all evidence points to this lump being benign and that the tests will be carried out later to confirm this, i.e. examination of the fluid and mammography.
4. Impress on her that the cyst is not malignant.
5. Impress on her that because she has had a cyst, this does not mean that she is more likely than anyone else to get a malignancy in her breast, but conversely, it does not mean that she is less likely to do so.
6. If at any time in the future she gets another lump it must not be assumed to be a cyst similar to this although that is the most likely diagnosis. It must be seen and treated immediately as an emergency as on this occasion to exclude any totally unrelated pathology having developed in the breast.

Post-operatively, the patient should be seen again in three weeks when the results will be through confirming the diagnosis and when an assessment can be made if the cyst is reforming.

Following this, if it has not reformed, she should be seen at three and then following six months' intervals impressing on her that if a lump develops she should not wait until the appointment comes up, but should get an appointment to be seen immediately.

★ ★ ★

Drainage of a hydrocele

A hydrocele presents as a scrotal swelling causing symptoms by its size and its weight. The fluid in the sac between the tunica albuginea and albicans causes the cystic swelling with the classical signs of a cystic swelling transilluminating with no cough impulse and the testis lying to the back of it and not underneath it.

The swelling transilluminates, is cystic on examination, and the cord above it can be palpated normally and once again it has no cough impulse or any evidence of being in communication with the peritoneal cavity.

The essential differential diagnosis is that of an irreducible hernia and if there is any doubt clinically then aspiration should be postponed.

Aspiration is advised and carried out for the following reasons:

(a) To ease symptoms,
(b) To be able to examine the fluid aspirated,
(c) To be able to palpate the testis underneath the hydrocele and exclude underlying pathology,
(d) In a small number of cases it may not refill so one aspiration could be adequate,
(e) In a further group of cases it may be the patient's wish to have repeated aspirations at intervals rather than be subjected to surgery,
(f) It may be that although surgery is contemplated eventually, repeated aspirations are a convenient way of controlling symtoms until that surgery can be arranged,
(g) If the patient is not fit for surgery.

Specific pre-operative treatment

The patient has to purchase and bring along a scrotal support with him on the day of operation.

Shaving is not usually necessary and a bath on the morning of the operation is sufficient.

Instruments

A Medicut needle
A large kidney dish
Large towelling set

Position on the table

Lying flat on the back with the legs splayed out.

Anaesthetic and surgical technique

The skin is cleaned with Savlon in water or Hibitane in water. Never use a spirit-based skin preparation.

Having cleaned the scrotum, appropriate towelling is arranged and the skin of the scrotum is stretched by the left hand over the hydrocele. Once this hydrocele and skin is grasped and tensed with the left hand that hand is not removed *under any circumstances* from that position until the aspiration is commenced.

The right hand then infiltrates a 1 cm diameter intra cutaneous injection of 2% Lignocaine with no Adrenaline, this usually arising in the skin or dartos layer.

After two minutes the needle, which has been withdrawn, is then inserted at right angles through the skin, through the centre part of the anaesthetised area and as it is slowly advanced towards the tense hydrocele so injection is carried out ahead of it.

Suddenly all the resistance to the injection will go as the sac is entered. The needle is then withdrawn and then after a minute, the Medicut needle is introduced in the same tract along the same line.

Once again there will be a 'give' as it enters the sac. It is then advanced a little and the stilette steel core of the needle is withdrawn about 1 cm and the combination then advanced again. Each time the stilette is withdrawn more as the needle with its sheath is advanced into the sac.

As it is a plastic, soft sheath, the end causes minimal damage to the inner layer of the sac should it impinge on it, as the last thing wanted is bleeding into the hydrocele fluid.

The inner trochar is now removed, the tension can be left off with the left hand and the syringe attached to the plastic cover then aspirates the hydrocele fluid.

Remember:

(a) To measure the total volume of fluid removed,
(b) To note the appearance,
(c) To send off at least 20 ccs for cytology examination for malignant cells and another specimen for culture,
(d) To palpate the testis at the end of the operation which is now able to be palpated due to the fluid being removed. If there is any doubt as to its normality an ultrasound examination should be arranged urgently.

Following the aspiration the plastic needle is removed, a small dressing is applied if necessary, and the patient advised to wear a scrotal support for two weeks, with as much rest as possible for the first 24 hours.

Post-operatively

Reassess after one week when the result of the cytology and the culture should be through and, if ultrasound has been necessary, this result will be also available. If all the tests are normal, the patient is referred back in six weeks for re-examination and assessment of any re-accumulation.

★ ★ ★

Catheterisation

Male catheterisation is usually carried out as an emergency for acute retention of urine caused by prostatic enlargement.

In the past, multiple strictures of GC origin were a diagnostic factor but now strictures are usually post-traumatic or iatrogenic.

The history of previous prostatic symptoms with recent precipitating causes, such as having to wait overlong to try to pass urine often associated with excessive alcohol intake, which tends rapidly to overfill the bladder and at the same time diminishes the urgency of response to the necessity to void.

There may be evidence of a chronic retention on to which an acute retention has developed.

The symptoms of the history combined with a painful, palpable tender bladder enlargement are diagnostic of the condition.

It is very much more preferable if catheterisation can be carried out as soon as possible to relieve the symptoms before referral to the local urological unit for further investigation and treatment.

Special documentation

Nil.

Shaving

Not necessary.

Surgical anatomy

The diameter of the urethra is said to be at its narrowest at the external meatus, thus implying that if a catheter goes past that site, it will pass the whole way up the urethra.

However, with the prostate swollen from its previous enlargement added to which is the oedema caused by straining and attempts at voiding, the prostatic urethra is tight but, despite this, can be stretched without physical damage.

Instruments

Balloon catheter of the Foley type of 18 gauge
Foley catheter introducer
Non-tooth forceps
1% Lignocaine Gel in a sterile tube
20 ml syringe
Water
Swabs
Kidney dish
Sterile spigot
Savlon for cleaning

Position

Flat on the back with legs splayed.

Surgical technique

The penis is cleaned with Savlon from the external meatus around the glans and shaft. The penis is first held with a sterile swab and the swab discarded after cleansing the glans. The glans is then held and the shaft cleaned.

With an uncircumcised patient, if the prepuce cannot be fully retracted, then the glans must be cleaned of smegma as well as possible.

The prepuce must not be dragged back if it is too tight as this might precipitate a phimosis on top of the original problem.

The towels are put on after cleaning and the kidney dish placed between the legs.

The sterile tube of Lignocaine 1% Gel which has been emptied from its packet on to the table then has its nozzle attached and a few drops of gel put just inside the external meatus and wiped around the surrounding glans.

Whilst this preparatory anaesthetic is working, the catheter is prepared by being emptied from its container and the balloon is tested by inflating with 20 ml of water.

This not only tests the balloon but also gives an impression to the surgeon of the tension needed to be applied on the syringe in order to inflate the balloon.

The outside of the catheter is lubricated with a little of the Lignocaine Gel 1%.

The Introducer is lubricated with a little of the Gel 1%.

The nozzle of the Lignocaine Gel is now inserted in the external meatus and the remaining contents of the tube of gel is squeezed into the penile urethra, squeezing the nozzle in the meatus with the left hand to stop it extravasating around the opening as the injection is made.

When all the gel has been squeezed in, the nozzle is removed and the urethra is squeezed by pressure with the left thumb on the frenulum region and the fingers on the glans.

The urethra is then stretched up a little and the swab held in the right hand is passed down the shaft from the glans milking the gel along the urethra around the external sphincter and into the prostatic urethra. The gel is kept in place for at least two minutes and it is essential to give it time to work before proceeding.

The catheter is now picked up with the forceps near its end and introduced into the meatus and urethra. It is pushed in with the forceps and when they reach the external meatus the catheter is held by pressure with the left thumb whilst a new grip on the catheter about 3 cms further back is taken with the forceps which then pushes it in that distance before the sequence is repeated.

The difficult and tight part is passing around the membranous urethra and through the prostatic urethra. However, slowly applying continuous pressure and easing it, with patience, usually succeeds.

Once in the bladder, the movement becomes easier but very occasionally the urine does not flow immediately. Quite often this is due to some of the gel in the tip of the catheter acting as a temporary block. Do not despair and do not remove the catheter. First push it in a little further to ensure that it is in the bladder, then, if necessary, clear it by milking the catheter or even injecting a little water up it.

When the urine starts to flow, let it empty a little before inflating the balloon, because a sudden inflation on a tense bladder causes quite considerable and unnecessary pain.

Let half the bladder empty quite rapidly into the kidney dish and then slow down the rate of emptying by using either a gate clip or by spigotting and unspiggoting the end of the catheter.

The introducer

If sustained pressure on the catheter has not been sufficient to enter the bladder round the membranous urethra and through the prostatic urethra, then the catheter should be removed and the introducer put into it. Before doing so, the introducer itself must be thoroughly lubricated.

It is vitally important to ensure that the tip of the introducer is at the end of the catheter and is kept there by the catheter being stretched and held stretched over the introducer all the time. If the catheter is not kept stretched over the introducer, the end of the introducer may pass through the top eye of the catheter and cause considerable damage to the urethra as an attempt is made to get the catheter into the bladder.

With the catheter stretched over the curved introducer and lubricated with gel, it is once again passed into the urethra and down to the external sphincter where it comes to a halt.

There, with the introducer curved upwards, the introducer and catheter over it is slowly angulated downwards which will bring the tip of the catheter through the external meatus and into the prostatic urethra.

No excessive force must be used as once the catheter tip with the introducer is through the external meatus, a firm downward rotation will ensure that the catheter passes through into the bladder without any further trouble.

It is then important to keep the catheter *in situ* whilst removing the introducer and this is done with a rotation movement the other way round as it is drawn out from the catheter.

From this point the management is the same.

Post-catheterisation

1. A catheter specimen of urine must be sent for immediate culture and analysis.
2. A referral to the genito-urinary unit should be made. The catheter in the meantime should be released and the bladder emptied by removing the spigot every four hours until that time.

★ ★ ★

Thrombosed external pile or peri-anal haematoma

Although blessed through years of usage as a thrombosed external pile, the condition referred to as such is very rarely a thrombosis in, but is rather a rupture from, a peri-anal vein lying in the peri-anal plexus.

The history is one of a sudden onset of severe pain in the peri-anal region followed by the appearance of a peri-anal lump, these symptoms are invariably associated with straining at defaecation.

The condition can be treated conservatively with rest, warm baths, analgesic, local anaesthetic and most important, suppositories to soften any formed mass in the rectum.

Alternatively, surgery can be advised which brings about an immediate relief of the acute pain.

Surgical anatomy

A peri-anal haematoma is a tense lump lying in the submucus and subcutaneous layer at the muco-cutaneous junction in the peri-anal region.

Special pre-operative treatment

Nil.

Instruments

A 15 small surgical scalpel
Cotton wool and swabs
2% Lignocaine Gel and 2% Lignocaine plain injection.

Position on the table

On the lateral side with the knees drawn up and the peri-anal haematoma on the under surface.

Anaesthetic

A cotton wool ball is firstly covered with half a tube of Lignocaine Gel and placed up against the external anal sphincter and against the surface of the peri-anal haematoma and is left there in place for five minutes.

Following cleansing, the 2% Lignocaine is very slowly injected with a fine needle under the surface of the skin and the mucosa over the peri-anal haemoatoma.

This injection must be slow as the pain in the haematoma is due to tension and the injection itself increases that tension before the anaesthetic can work.

It is very rarely that one has to use more than ½ cc of 2% Lignocaine injection after which the needle is removed.

Surgical technique

The area is cleaned with Savlon — no spirit-based preparation should be used.

The gloved index finger of the left hand is lubricated with the remaining 2% Lignocaine Gel and slowly inserted rectally. This then enables the thumb of the left hand to be used to steady the peri-anal haematoma on the sphincter side.

The haematoma is incised radially. On incision of the covering layers, the haematoma will then shell out very easily.

This may be accompanied by some vascular oozing and this is allowed to drain through the operative site which, because it remains open, stops any further tension recurring and the condition recurring.

Half-strength Eusol dressings seem to be as comfortable as any to be used.

Post-operative

The next day the patient is encouraged to take baths and if he has not had a bowel action further glycerin suppositories are given to try to ensure that the first bowel action when it occurs is not constipated.

Post-operative management

1. Relating to the surgery — baths, social dressings of half-strength Eusol and analgesics as necessary until healing has taken place.
2. When healing has taken place, the patient must have a full history, rectal examination, proctoscopy and sigmoidoscopy carried out to ensure that there is no underlying predisposing cause which led to the straining, constipation and onset of the peri-anal haematoma. This examination is essential and mandatory, and it must be stressed to the patient how important it is for this to be done.

CHAPTER 13

Post-operative complications and treatment

Despite having taken all the care possible in the performance of any operation and having carried out the procedure with expertise and diligence, any surgical procedure is at risk of developing post-operative complications.

Complications can broadly be classified into those which are liable to occur with any operation, and those which may occur relating to the specific operation which are unique to it. These latter complications will be discussed in the chapter on the specific operation.

Complications related to the anaesthetic administered are dealt with elsewhere.

Haemorrhage

By far the most common post-operative complication in the immediate post-operative period is haemorrhage. Bleeding occurs when a ligature, which has been tied around a vessel, slips before the vessel has closed off its lumen with clot and so starts to bleed again.

This slip is quite often associated with movement at the end of the operation, or is perhaps due to the blood pressure in the vessel rising and causing it to slip. Alternatively, it could be due to a poorly tied ligature.

The bleeding of fresh red blood causes a swelling which can be associated with visible bleeding through the incision.

An assessment of the depth of the bleeding must be made. The combination of swelling with a little visible bleeding means probably the problem is a deep level, whereas bleeding visibly with less swelling means it would probably be coming from the skin edge.

The immediate treatment is pressure, and if the operative site is a limb it is necessary to combine the pressure with elevation.

If the skin edge is bleeding, pressure for four to five minutes followed by a slow release of the pressure is sometimes adequate. Otherwise, if the site of the skin edge bleeding point can be identified, a skin stitch can be put in to under-run the bleeding point and so control it when tied.

Deep bleeding is more difficult. Pressure will control it initially and if it has stopped, then a deep collection is left. This is very liable to get further complications at a later date, such as becoming infected or discharging itself through the incision, thus spoiling the scar.

Small collections can be left alone, but with anything of any size it is well worthwhile trying to aspirate it. This is done by cleaning the skin site and introducing a needle through the incision between the skin edges where this can be carried out painlessly.

If the blood cannot be aspirated then it is well worthwhile taking a stitch or two out, evacuating the blood and clot there and then, securing the bleeding point if it is still spurting, and re-sewing up.

This does not entail 'loss of face' as it happens to everyone in the best regulated circles, but what it does mean is that the healing will progress normally and a good result will be obtained, whereas if a haematoma is left it may well cause problems later.

Haematoma

A haematoma tends to develop slowly in the later part of the post-operative period probably by oozing into a dead space which has not been obliterated correctly during the operation.

It presents as a swelling, but this swelling is due to a clot and it cannot be aspirated until that clot liquefies. In the meantime it is very liable to become infected and if so it has to be treated as an abscess. If it does not get infected when it has liquified it can be aspirated.

If the needle, after cleaning the skin, is introduced through the incision it is painless and the patient does not even feel the prick.

When the old blood has been removed, a pressure dressing helps to close the cavity and stop any further accumulation, although the walls of the cavity at that point are in fact a fibrin clot.

Infection

Cellulitis

Cellulitis is a superficial infection around the operative incision indicated by redness, oedema, and a spreading cellulitis associated with an elevated temperature in the early post-operative phase.

This is probably due to infection at the operation and is an indication for the exhibition of a wide-spectrum antibiotic in a high dosage combined with rest of the part.

As this is a cellulitis there is at the time no collection of pus so there is no necessity to drain the area. If it does localise superficially it becomes known as a stitch abscess and removal of the relevant stitch will effect drainage.

Abscess

An abscess is usually due to an infected deep haematoma. This develops later and presents as a tender, throbbing lump, usually under the scar. The patient will have a raised temperature, and there will be oedema of the skin over the lump where it has started to 'point'.

This site of pointing, if surgery has been undertaken, is usually under the scar and the first line of treatment is drainage. This is achieved by removing one or two stitches. The pus is encouraged to discharge by easing the skin edges apart at that position with the point of a sterile needle or a little gentle traction.

If this is not successful then a little local heat, rather like the old-time poultice, will bring the abscess to a head and it will discharge.

If the abscess is large and it is envisaged that it will have to discharge for a few days, then the skin edge will have to be encouraged to stay open: the best drain to achieve this is provided by cutting off the finger of a sterile glove and tucking it into the gap.

Always put a safety pin through the part of the drain outside the patient to prevent it slipping into the cavity.

There is usually no indication for antibiotic treatment in the case of an abscess which has been adequately drained unless there is an associated cellulitis, or the temperature does not drop following the drainage.

Sinus

After drainage of an abscess or its natural discharge through the incision, the discharge may continue and then the situation has changed from an abscess draining into a sinus which is defined as a granulation tissue-lined tract opening on an epithelial lined surface.

This sinus will usually close as the abscess deep down drains, but if it continues for an abnormally long time, it probably implies that there is a foreign body deep down in the abscess cavity. This may be a foreign body introduced at the time of trauma or a foreign body introduced at the time of surgery, the most common of which is a stitch.

As all deep stitches and ties in the operations described are carried out with absorbable material, the part that is last to absorb is the knot. Therefore, given time, the sinus should close with the discharge of a knot of the absorbable stitch, and time is the main essence of the treatment. However, if there is a foreign body that has not been cleared out before, this may have to be explored subsequently.

Antibiotics locally or generally have no place in the treatment of this sinus.

If the epithelium of the skin grows down into the sinus tract it has reached a chronic stage and will probably need further delineation with a sinogram, and referred to a surgical colleague for exploration and further treatment.

Dehiscence

Very occasionally the incision may have been sewn up under tension. This is to be avoided if at all possible, but if it has been necessary a stitch may either pull through or, if not tied, become loose. If the incision is clean, it may be able to be supported by a strap as the other stitches are in place. If not, it may have to be replaced. This can be done under a little local anaesthetic introduced via a needle through the gap the dehiscence has caused, so being painless for the patient.

Complications needing more extensive treatment

The most immediate complication is one of severe bleeding. If there has been any severe bleeding very, very occasionally the patient may need monitoring after the bleeding has been controlled for a period. If this is necessary the patient may need admission as an emergency to hospital.

Late complications

Recurrence

Whatever the original reason for the surgery, the condition may recur, or what was originally thought to be a benign condition may come back, following histological examination, as malignant.

In these cases there is no justification to return and try to do further surgery with the facilities and the expertise that are available. Any further surgery is, by definition, bound to be more extensive and, by definition also, because it is a recurrence and more extensive it is bound to be more difficult, and for these reasons should be carried out by a specialist surgeon. He will have the facility for operating under general anaesthetic where the operative conditions are much better if he so needs.

It is, therefore, manifestly important to keep a good rapport with surgical colleagues at the local hospital and to keep all lines of communication open just in case this eventuality arises, which on pure statistical grounds, it may well do.

Deep infection or chronic sinus

A deep abscess or a chronic sinus may develop if there has been inadequate drainage or if there is a residual foreign body present.

This needs radiological delineation and may need further exploring either under a general anaesthetic, or with a tourniquet etc. and in most cases, once again, this is a later complication which should be referred to the local consultant surgeon.

Keloid formation

If a bad scar results post-operatively either because it has developed keloid, which was not suspected from the pre-operative history or because, for example, it was not sited quite correctly as the dictates of the surgery had made the choice of selection limited, then there are two things that should be done.

1. Do not rush into any precipitant action or give the patient the impression urgent action is required, as time is on your side. Scar tissue will contract and become paler and the problem will become more defined.
2. In either case, whether a Z-plasty revision of the scar may be needed for a poor scar or a post-operative treatment to try to reduce keloid, this is best performed by a specialist and once again may need a general anaesthetic or tourniquet, etc. and perhaps, in this context, a plastic surgical colleague might be the one whose help to seek.

As has been discussed before in the history taking, the possibility of keloid formation might have been picked up, but it is very difficult to do Z-plasties of any extent and revising scars without considerable expertise under local anaesthetic.

Other complications which occur after more major surgery or surgery under general anaesthetic, such as deep vein thrombosis, pulmonary emboli, pulmonary infections and collapse, etc. are all very unusual in the context of minor surgery under local anaesthetic, and will not be discussed here.

Appendix: Surgical equipment suppliers

Instruments

Downs Surgical Ltd
Parkway Industrial Estate
Sheffield S9 4WJ

Charles F. Thackray Ltd
Shire Oak Street
Leeds LS6 2DP

Codman Ltd
110–112 High Street
Marlow
Bucks SL6 1QO

Senard Medical Ltd
131 Great Suffolk Street
London SE1 1PP

Lester Surgical
28 Delauneys Road
Crumpsall
Manchester M8 6QS
(will also supply inexpensive tables and lamps)

Gloves

Regent Gloves
LRC Products Ltd
London E4 8QA

Sutures

Ethicon Ltd
Bankhead Avenue
Edinburgh EH11 4HE

Caps and masks

Surgikos
Kirkton Campus
Livingston
W. Lothian EH54 78AT

Sterilizer

Little Sister—Mark 3 (works off 15amp plug)
Eschmann & Walsh Ltd
Peter Road
Lancing
W. Sussex BN15 8TJ

Dressing packs

Smith & Nephew Medical Ltd
81 Hessle Road
Hull HU3 2BN

Johnson & Johnson
Coronation Road
Ascot
Berks SL5 9EY

Molnlycke Ltd
Southfields Road
Dunstable
Bedfordshire LU6 3ET

INDEX